Exemplary Social Intervention Programs for Members and Their Families

The *Marriage & Family Review* series:

- *Cults and the Family*, edited by Florence Kaslow and Marvin B. Sussman
- *Alternatives to Traditional Family Living*, edited by Harriet Gross and Marvin B. Sussman
- *Intermarriage in the United States*, edited by Gary A. Crester and Joseph J. Leon
- *Family Systems and Inheritance Patterns*, edited by Judith N. Cates and Marvin B. Sussman
- *The Ties that Bind: Men's and Women's Social Networks*, edited by Laura Lein and Marvin B. Sussman
- *Social Stress and the Family: Advances and Developments in Family Stress Theory and Research*, edited by Hamilton I. McCubbin, Marvin B. Sussman, and Joan M. Patterson
- *Human Sexuality and the Family*, edited by James W. Maddock, Gerhard Neubeck, and Marvin B. Sussman
- *Obesity and the Family*, edited by David J. Kallen and Marvin B. Sussman
- *Women and the Family*, edited by Beth B. Hess and Marvin B. Sussman
- *Personal Computers and the Family*, edited by Marvin B. Sussman
- *Pets and the Family*, edited by Marvin B. Sussman
- *Families and the Energy Transition*, edited by John Byrne, David A. Schulz, and Marvin B. Sussman
- *Men's Changing Roles in the Family*, edited by Robert A. Lewis and Marvin B. Sussman
- *The Charybdis Complex: Redemption of Rejected Marriage and Family Journal Articles*, edited by Marvin B. Sussman
- *Families and the Prospect of Nuclear Attack/Holocaust*, edited by Teresa D. Marciano and Marvin B. Sussman
- *Family Medicine: The Maturing of a Discipline*, edited by William J. Doherty, Charles E. Christianson, and Marvin B. Sussman
- *Childhood Disability and Family Systems*, edited by Michael Ferrari and Marvin B. Sussman
- *Alternative Health Maintenance and Healing Systems for Families*, edited by Doris Y. Wilkinson and Marvin B. Sussman
- *Deviance and the Family*, edited by Frank E. Hagan and Marvin B. Sussman
- *Transitions to Parenthood*, edited by Rob Palkovitz and Marvin B. Sussman
- *AIDS and Families: Report of the AIDS Task Force Groves Conference on Marriage and the Family*, edited by Eleanor D. Macklin
- *Museum Visits and Activities for Family Life Enrichment*, edited by Barbara H. Butler and Marvin B. Sussman
- *Cross-Cultural Perspectives on Families, Work, and Change*, edited by Katja Boh, Giovanni Sgritta, and Marvin B. Sussman
- *Homosexuality and Family Relations*, edited by Frederick W. Bozett and Marvin B. Sussman

- *Families in Community Settings: Interdisciplinary Perspectives*, edited by Donald G. Unger and Marvin B. Sussman
- *Corporations, Businesses, and Families*, edited by Roma S. Hanks and Marvin B. Sussman
- *Families: Intergenerational and Generational Connections*, edited by Susan K. Pfeifer and Marvin B. Sussman
- *Wider Families: New Traditional Family Forms*, edited by Teresa D. Marciano and Marvin B. Sussman
- *Publishing in Journals on the Family: A Survey and Guide for Scholars, Practitioners, and Students*, edited by Roma S. Hanks, Linda Matocha, and Marvin B. Sussman
- *Publishing in Journals on the Family: Essays on Publishing*, edited by Roma S. Hanks, Linda Matocha, and Marvin B. Sussman
- *American Families and the Future: Analyses of Possible Destinies*, edited by Barbara H. Settles, Roma S. Hanks, and Marvin B. Sussman
- *Families on the Move: Migration, Immigration, Emigration, and Mobility*, edited by Barbara H. Settles, Daniel E. Hanks III, and Marvin B. Sussman
- *Single Parent Families: Diversity, Myths and Realities*, edited by Shirley M. H. Hanson, Marsha L. Heims, Doris J. Julian, and Marvin B. Sussman
- *Exemplary Social Intervention Programs for Members and Their Families*, edited by David Guttmann and Marvin B. Sussman

Exemplary Social Intervention Programs for Members and Their Families

David Guttmann
Marvin B. Sussman
Editors

The Haworth Press, Inc.
New York · London · Norwood (Australia)

Exemplary Social Intervention Programs for Members and Their Families has also been published as *Marriage & Family Review,* Volume 21, Numbers 1/2 1995.

Paperback edition published in 1997.

Cover design by Stephanie Torta.

Library of Congress Cataloging-in-Publication Data

Exemplary social intervention programs for members and their families / David Guttmann, Marvin B. Sussman, editors.

    p.   cm.

    Includes bibliographical references.

    ISBN 0-7890-0214-0 (alk. paper)

    1. Social service–United States–Case studies. 2. Evaluation research (Social action programs)–United States. I. Guttmann, David. II. Sussman, Marvin B.

HV91.E95 1994

362'.0425–dc20   94-30137

                                                CIP

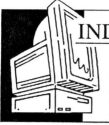

INDEXING & ABSTRACTING

Contributions to this publication are selectively indexed or abstracted in print, electronic, online, or CD-ROM version(s) of the reference tools and information services listed below. This list is current as of the copyright date of this publication. See the end of this section for additional notes.

- *Abstracts in Social Gerontology: Current Literature on Aging,* National Council on the Aging, Library, 409 Third Street SW, 2nd Floor, Washington, DC 20024

- *Abstracts of Research in Pastoral Care & Counseling,* Loyola College, 7135 Minstrel Way, Suite 101, Columbia, MD 21045

- *Academic Abstracts/CD-ROM,* EBSCO Publishing, P.O. Box 2250, Peabody, MA 01960-7250

- *AGRICOLA Database,* National Agricultural Library, 10301 Baltimore Boulevard, Room 002, Beltsville, MD 20705

- *Applied Social Sciences Index & Abstracts (ASSIA) (Online: ASSI via Data-Star) (CDRom: ASSIA Plus),* Bowker-Saur Limited, Maypole House, Maypole Road, East Grinstead, West Sussex RH19 1HH, England

- *Current Contents: Social & Behavioral Sciences (CC/S&BS) (weekly Table of Contents Service), and Social Science Citation Index. Articles also searchable through Social SciSearch, ISI's online database and in ISI's Research Alert current awareness service,* Institute for Scientific Information, 3501 Market Street, Philadelphia, PA 19104-3302 (USA)

- *Family Life Educator "Abstracts Section",* ETR Associates, P.O. Box 1830, Santa Cruz, CA 95061-1830

- *Family Violence & Sexual Assault Bulletin,* Family Violence & Sexual Assault Institute, 1310 Clinic Drive, Tyler, TX 75701

- *Guide to Social Science & Religion in Periodical Literature,* National Periodical Library, P.O. Box 3278, Clearwater, FL 34630

- *Index to Periodical Articles Related to Law,* University of Texas, 727 East 26th Street, Austin, TX 78705

- *Inventory of Marriage and Family Literature (online and hard copy),* National Council on Family Relations, 3989 Central Avenue NE, Suite 550, Minneapolis, MN 55421

(continued)

- *PASCAL International Bibliography T205: Sciences de l'information Documentation,* INIST/CNRS-Service Gestion des Documents Primaires, 2, allee du Parc de Brabois, F-54514 Vandoeuvre-les-Nancy, Cedex, France

- *Periodical Abstracts, Research I (general & basic reference indexing & abstracting data-base from University Microfilms International (UMI), 300 North Zeeb Road, PO Box 1346, Ann Arbor, MI 48106-1346),* UMI Data Courier, P.O. Box 32770, Louisville, KY 40232-2770

- *Periodical Abstracts, Research II (broad coverage indexing & abstracting data-base from University Microfilms International (UMI), 300 North Zeeb Road, PO Box 1346, Ann Arbor, MI 48106-1346),* UMI Data Courier, P.O. Box 32770, Louisville, KY 40232-2770

- *Population Index,* Princeton University Office Population, 21 Prospect Avenue, Princeton, NJ 08544-2091

- *Psychological Abstracts (PsycINFO),* American Psychological Association, P.O. Box 91600, Washington, DC 20090-1600

- *Sage Family Studies Abstracts (SFSA),* Sage Publications, Inc., 2455 Teller Road, Newbury Park, CA 91320

- *Social Planning/Policy & Development Abstracts (SOPODA),* Sociological Abstracts, Inc., P.O. Box 22206, San Diego, CA 92192-0206

- *Social Sciences Index (from Volume 1 & continuing),* The H.W. Wilson Company, 950 University Avenue, Bronx, NY 10452

- *Social Work Abstracts,* National Association of Social Workers, 750 First Street NW, 8th Floor, Washington, DC 20002

- *Sociological Abstracts (SA),* Sociological Abstracts, Inc., P.O. Box 22206, San Diego, CA 92192-0206

- *Special Educational Needs Abstracts,* Carfax Information Systems, P.O. Box 25, Abingdon, Oxfordshire OX14 3UE, United Kingdom

- *Studies on Women Abstracts,* Carfax Publishing Company, P.O. Box 25, Abingdon, Oxfordshire OX14 3UE, United Kingdom

- *Violence and Abuse Abstracts: A Review of Current Literature on Interpersonal Violence (VAA),* Sage Publications, Inc., 2455 Teller Road, Newbury Park, CA 91320

(continued)

SPECIAL BIBLIOGRAPHIC NOTES

related to special journal issues (separates)
and indexing/abstracting

❑ indexing/abstracting services in this list will also cover material in any "separate" that is co-published simultaneously with Haworth's special thematic journal issue or DocuSerial. Indexing/abstracting usually covers material at the article/chapter level.

❑ monographic co-editions are intended for either non-subscribers or libraries which intend to purchase a second copy for their circulating collections.

❑ monographic co-editions are reported to all jobbers/wholesalers/approval plans. The source journal is listed as the "series" to assist the prevention of duplicate purchasing in the same manner utilized for books-in-series.

❑ to facilitate user/access services all indexing/abstracting services are encouraged to utilize the co-indexing entry note indicated at the bottom of the first page of each article/chapter/contribution.

❑ this is intended to assist a library user of any reference tool (whether print, electronic, online, or CD-ROM) to locate the monographic version if the library has purchased this version but not a subscription to the source journal.

❑ individual articles/chapters in any Haworth publication are also available through the Haworth Document Delivery Services (HDDS).

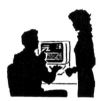

Exemplary Social Intervention Programs for Members and Their Families

CONTENTS

ABOUT THE EDITORS

David Guttmann, DSW, is a former Dean and currently Professor in the School of Social Work, Haifa University, Israel. He received his Doctor of Social Work Degree from Catholic University of America in 1974, at which time he joined the faculty of Catholic University, then leaving that post to join the Haifa faculty in 1987. He is an international expert on Logo Therapy, working closely with its founder, Viktor E. Frankl, in conceptualizing and applying this approach to individual and family issues and problems. His scholarly work focuses on the aged and families and the utility of such research knowledge for social work practice.

Marvin B. Sussman, PhD, is UNIDEL Professor of Human Behavior Emeritus at the College of Human Resources, University of Delaware: and Member of the CORE Faculty, Union Graduate School, Union Institute, Cincinnati, Ohio. A member of many professional organizations, he was awarded the 1980 Ernest W. Burgess Award of the National Council on Family Relations. In 1983, he was elected to the prestigious academy of Groves for scholarly contributions to the field, as well as awarded a life-long membership for services to the Groves Conference on Marriage and the Family in 1984. Dr. Sussman received the Distinguished Family Scholar Award of the Society for the Study of Social Problems (1985) and the Lee Founders Award (1992), SSSP most prestigious Professional Award. Also, in 1992, he was the recipient of the State of Delaware Gerontological Society Award for contributions to research and education in the family and aging fields. Dr. Sussman has published over 250 articles and books on family, community, rehabilitation, organizations, health and aging.

Introduction

David Guttmann
Marvin B. Sussman

"Making a difference" is a prerequisite of a moral society. Hence, it is a desired goal in most societies. In socialization, nurturance, and training of the young, making a difference, if not openly promulgated, is an implied expectation. All the hard work in school and related activities is intended to develop one's competencies to benefit oneself, family, and the larger society.

On another level, many individuals are unsung heroes–heroes who serve others who are unrecognized and seek no benefits for their actions. They are like the elderly gentleman walking along an isolated beach covered with hundreds of starfish washed ashore during a tumultuous storm. Every few steps he would stoop with difficulty, pick up one and toss it back into the ocean. A young lad was watching and began to follow the man. His curiosity was so profound that he ran up to the man and said, "Hey Mister, what are you doing? There are hundreds of starfish, look. You can't help them, it makes no difference to throw one back into the water." The gent replied with a laugh as he stooped, picked up a starfish and flung it into the water, "It makes a difference to this one!"

Human societies have countless members who with quiet and unassuming demeaners march to serve others. Their work enhances the goodness, a much needed and desired attribute of a quality society. The person who makes a difference, acts for others in goodness, is likely to have the virtues of altruism, responsibility, justice, ega-

[Haworth co-indexing entry note]: "Introduction." Guttmann, David, and Marvin B. Sussman. Co-published simultaneously in *Marriage & Family Review* (The Haworth Press, Inc.) Vol. 21, No. 1/2, 1995, pp. 1-7; and: *Exemplary Social Intervention Programs for Members and Their Families* (ed: David Guttmann, and Marvin B. Sussman) The Haworth Press, Inc., 1995, pp. 1-7. Multiple copies of this article/chapter may be purchased from The Haworth Document Delivery Center [1-800-3-HA-WORTH; 9:00 a.m. - 5:00 p.m. (EST)].

litarianism, and honesty (Nicholas, 1994). Making a difference is not limited to the perceptions, feelings, and actions of individuals. Organizations can hold in their myths and beliefs and function in their practices the virtues of goodness.

The virtues of goodness can be found in the actions, beliefs and myths of organizations. In a coherent and coordinated manner such systems function to make a difference for whom they serve. Such organizations can be viewed as possessing exemplary programs which are prototypes of best and innovative practice and marked for widespread dissemination and utilization. In many instances program developers were risk takers, deviating from traditional modes and practices, derided by professional peers. The steadfast belief that they and their organization could improve the workplace, service to the client and society resulted in actions of heroic proportions. The virtues of goodness, universally expressed, guided the process and outcomes so salutatory that it is appropriate to label such organizations as exemplary.

In this special volume the editors have selected a number of organizations and individuals whose stories fit an exemplary paradigm and which are worthwhile to report and disseminate.

A popular belief is that disabled adults cannot and should not care for their well-bodied and well-minded children. It is believed that families who have disabled or chronically ill children or youth need primarily professional services which are their main source of support and treatment. The disability independent living movement disavows this myopic perception of reality. Megan Kirshbaum, in the article "Serving Families with Disability Issues," indicates how the *Through the Looking Glass* organization provides clinical and supportive services, training, and research involving families where an adult with a disability or medical condition takes responsibility for the care of well-functioning children. Children who are disabled or chronically ill are cared for by adults in this learning community. Provision of services in a traditional manner is not an adequate description of what the work of the Looking Glass staff does. They involve family members as copartners in support, caring, and rehabilitative activities. The Looking Glass is a transforming organization demonstrating that creative, innovative, and risk-taking ideas and actions can make a difference. Disabled and chronically ill adults and children can continue to live in family homes as a consequence of their own tireless efforts with support from concerned and nurturing professionals.

Zev Harel, in his paper "Serving Holocaust Survivors and Survivor Families," does not present an exemplary intervention program, but one is implied. Sensitivity of professionals in working with holocaust victims is a cardinal prerequisite. Special understanding is required of recent non-pathologically oriented research on the effects of stress on social and psychological well-being in later life. In recognizing that survivors of the Holocaust are not a homogenous group but express diversity in personality, perception of reality, memory of trauma and loss and control of stress, the professional has the beginnings of an intervention strategy for treatment of older survivors experiencing extreme stress.

Craig Whitman's article, "Heading Toward Normal: Deinstitutionalization for the Mentally Retarded Client," is his story of being an adult developmental home provider for two mentally retarded individuals. These two persons, Thomas and Lenny, lived semi-independently in a house next door to the author's. Craig Whitman, a social worker, says, "During this time, I have attempted to intervene in ways that promote personal growth and greater independence for my clients. Each man has responded in his own unique ways by reflecting more competence and greater enjoyment of a lifestyle typically not available to mentally retarded people who are participants in the social services system. The opportunity to witness Lenny and Thomas' growth has been very meaningful to me as I feel that the place of the social worker in this consciously created lifestyle. . . ."

Whitman's experience can be classified as a "make a difference" phenomenon. The process he describes is both empowering and nurturing. It is removed from the extremes of keeping the mentally retarded incarcerated in institutions or "dumping" them into the streets of their home communities. The process recognizes the semi-independent status of the mentally retarded and the variability of such individuals in movement to a higher independent state.

The Mueller and Patton paper titled "Working with Poor Families–Lessons Learned from Practice" is a report on ". . . the diverse experiences and evaluations of seven effective parenting/family stability programs which were part of the McKnight Foundation's Families in Poverty (FIP) initiative." Successful programs experienced high levels of exchange of information, sensitivity to the unique needs of both client families and practitioners, a resonated agency mission clearly understood by the serving professionals and client families, and goodness behavior. Goodness consists of altruism, responsibility, egalitarianism, justice, and honesty (op. cit.).

In the United States and abroad caring and assisting multiproblem families on the journey to independence has been a continuous endeavor. Sharlin and Shamai, in their article "Intervention with Families in Extreme Distress (FED)," provide an Israeli experience. In a well-constructed pilot empirical study aimed to break the cycle of poverty of distressed families they derive an intervention model. This model requires a team of dedicated professionals who can deal with the intrafamily power dynamics and the normative demands of organizations and institutions outside the family. A holistic family approach in working with families experiencing distress is evident. The intervention strategies suggest that they are making a difference for the FED. Longitudinal research with a larger number of families and social work personnel is indicated in order to evaluate the efficacy of current intervention practices.

We tend to view "making a difference" in a positive light vis-à-vis the starfish story presented in the beginning of this "Introduction." Yet, interventions which plan to make a positive difference in the lives of individuals may have negative consequences. Ruth Landau, in her article "The Impact of New Medical Technologies in Human Reproduction on Children's Personal Safety and Well-Being in the Family," raises this issue of child abuse by uncontrolled and largely unregulated medical technologies. Our myth that scientific advances have an endemic goodness obscures the risks to the child's and other family members' well-being. Dr. Landau indicates in a compelling manner how a child's well-being can be affected by the circumstances of conception. Treatment and ethical issues and what are the best interests of children are considered. To make a positive difference may call for a new paradigm on how these advancing medical technologies are to be used in the best interest of the child and other family members and those of medical scientists.

The continuing high incidence of first marriage dissolutions and companionate remarriage has resulted in an ever-increasing prevalence of stepfamilies. Today this family form is often called the blended family. This name invokes the image of homogeneity, a proper mix of elements. One intention was undoubtedly to counteract the historic denigration of the stepfamily as a situation where children are neglected and abused by the nonputative parent. The Cinderella and Hansel and Gretel stories epitomize the wicked stepparent.

Regardless of its history, stepfamily members often experience inordinate stress because of ambiguities regarding correct interpersonal relationships, appropriate boundaries for the expression of intimacy and role expectations. Donald Fausel examines these issues and goes beyond normal intellectual discourse. He states the issue, how can one reduce the high stress experienced by step-couples by achieving and using new coping skills. He then proceeds to do an empirical test involving stepcouples in Stress Inoculation Training (SIT) initially developed by Donald Meichenbaum (1985) and operationalized and tested by Professor Fausel, using a training handbook he developed.

The intervention program appears to make a difference. Stepcouples report that they experience less stress as a consequence of the program. To go beyond clinical validity a more controlled experimental study is indicated. Sufficient work has been done to date to warrant a longitudinal study on causality, to firmly establish if such a program reduces stress significantly and the maintenance of the reduction over time.

In the article on Pilgrimage by Kris Jeter a story unfolds. In part, it is the tale of Kris Ayalla Jeter and, in part, the journey of many others on pilgrimages from time immemorial.

The author indicates that human service professionals have not utilized this process in treatment and thus have lost a viable ally in rebuilding the family's structure and interpersonal relations and in treating emotionally and mentally ill individuals. By ignoring or neglecting this powerful process to maintain one's psychic and spiritual well-being, the possibilities to go beyond treatment to reform oppressive social conditions are severely compromised.

The opportunity to become a social artist of change is now possible by incorporating components of the pilgrimage paradigm in one's practice. Dr. Jeter, in her essay, provides case studies and rationales for pilgrimages, their meaning and significance to the participants, and the strong bonding which results among both family and nonfamily members as a consequence of their participation. Rooted in history, the pilgrimage today provides what it did in the past: respite care, healing, spiritual awakening and development, social interaction, and great potential for social reform. Dr. Jeter demonstrates how human service professionals, particularly social workers can "make a difference" by incorporating the pilgrimage process into their armory of treatment techniques and skills.

In review, a human service program to be characterized as exemplary, something different from the ordinary, one that makes a difference, has to enchant the reviewer with its unique characteristics and processes. In all likelihood, the program creators have adopted a new paradigm, a new way of perceiving and viewing observable phenomena. The program developers earnestly believe that the old way of providing services is not working optimally. In some instances it has negative effects upon those they do or intend to serve.

Other conditions and intentions provoke efforts to create exemplary human service programs. Change is considered by society watchers as one of the few constants. You can always count on change to occur. Thus, efforts to keep up with modifications in values, ideologies, beliefs, institutional policies and practices requires modifications, even cosmetic ones, in service delivery. For those who go beyond cosmetic changes there is the opportunity to do a traditionectomy, moving to a new model of service buttressed by new values, ideologies, myths and practices.

Related to the change phenomenon and the search for improved models of service is the takeover of organizations by new leaders. The expectations are explicit or implied that the old ways will be modified or eliminated. New paradigms of structure and processes emerge. Some are second order change with drastic reorganization of goals and means to deliver services while others are cosmetic. Those who adopt new paradigms with its endemic new values, archetypes, myths, and ideologies will do things in novel and creative ways. They will be the social artists who will "make a difference."

REFERENCES

Meichenbaum, Donald (1994). Stress Inoculation Training. NY: Pergamon Press.
Nicholas, Mary (1994). The Mystery of Goodness. Evanston, IL: W.W. Horton & Co., Inc.

Serving Families with Disability Issues: Through the Looking Glass

Megan Kirshbaum

SUMMARY. The article describes an agency, Through the Looking Glass, which has provided peer-oriented clinical and supportive services, professional training, and research serving infants, young children and families with a disability or medical issue. Historical context is provided regarding disability issues relevant to the program's mission and philosophy. The evolution of the agency is outlined. A theoretical framework is illustrated with clinical anecdotes.

INTRODUCTION

Through the Looking Glass is a non-profit organization in Berkeley, California which since 1982 has pioneered peer-oriented clinical and supportive services, professional training, and research serving infants, young children and families with a disability or medical issue. The roots of the program are in the disability independent living movement. Therefore a brief disability history pro-

Address correspondence to Megan Kirshbaum, Executive Director, Through the Looking Glass, 801 Peralta Avenue, Berkeley, CA 94707.

The described work was supported in part by the Easter Seal Research Foundation, the Regional Center of the East Bay, United Way, and in particular by the National Institute on Disability and Rehabilitation Research, U.S. Department of Education.

[Haworth co-indexing entry note]: "Serving Families with Disability Issues: Through the Looking Glass." Kirshbaum, Megan. Co-published simultaneously in *Marriage & Family Review* (The Haworth Press, Inc.) Vol. 21, No. 1/2, 1995, pp. 9-28; and: *Exemplary Social Intervention Programs for Members and Their Families* (ed: David Guttmann, and Marvin B. Sussman) The Haworth Press, Inc., 1995, pp. 9-28. Multiple copies of this article/chapter may be purchased from The Haworth Document Delivery Center [1-800-3-HAWORTH; 9:00 a.m. - 5:00 p.m. (EST)].

vides a framework which informs the mission and evolution of the organization.

DISABILITY CONTEXT

It is helpful to recall the situation at the outset of the disability movement. Unlike people of color or people from different ethnic groups whose communities and families provide pride and identity that helps compensate for the overall stigma and oppression, the overwhelming majority of people with disabilities had no such group culture. The most notable exception was the deaf community, which provided a relatively strong sense of cultural identity. Groupings were traditionally defined according to able-bodied professionals' disease and disability categories, e.g., the Multiple Sclerosis Society and the United Cerebral Palsy Association. Language reinforced this, referring to a person as the quadriplegic, the CP–defining people by pathologies rather than as individuals who happen to have disabilities. Even the achievements of these pathology cluster people were portrayed as exceptions, overcompensations and inspirations. In reaction, the disability independent living movement, the civil rights movement for people with disabilities, began to develop. Organizing around common social needs, a sense of culture began to emerge in these disability communities. Initially, many of the organizations were reacting to the way life had been defined by the patient role. They emphasized crossing medically defined disability lines in order to enhance clout, and emphasized independence, empowerment and respect for fully participating adult members of society rather than dependent roles. They stressed that the person with a disability is an expert on his or her disability, is a provider, and not just a recipient of services.

When one works with a person impacted by this emerging disability culture one is frequently doing cross-cultural therapy. There is variation in the degree to which any individual with a disability participates in a disability community or has a conscious sense of cultural identification. Yet, the personal intensity of disability experience and the commonality of social oppression frequently result in ties between those with personal disability experience, in contrast to those without such experience. An able-bodied therapist working with a client with a disability may be in a position that is comparable to a Caucasian therapist working with a client who is African-American.

Sensitivity regarding the medical model is particularly common in the disability culture(s). It is helpful to recall the connotation of the medical realm and therefore the especial importance of services that respect autonomy and personhood and that avoid pathologizing. The medical realm often has a charged personal psychological meaning for a person with a disability and his or her family members. There has often been a cumulative history of multiple traumatic medical events in childhood and/or adulthood. There is also often a history of professionals underestimating the reactive impact of the trauma, with a consequential psychological pathologizing of people with disabilities and their families.

Prior to the founding of Through the Looking Glass there was a startling gulf in society between the realms of adults with disabilities and infants with disabilities. This separation was manifest on the personal level of families as well as among professionals. Conferences which focused on infants with disabilities reflected no awareness of the lives of adults with disabilities. Indeed, the conferences failed to include such individuals. It was as if infants with disabilities had no futures.

The "fix it" orientation pervades most interventions with children who have disabilities. The focus on ameliorating deficits or pathologies often results in making a child feel broken, fragmented, and dehumanized. Anne and H. Rutherford Turnbull articulated this issue in their article, "Stepping Back from Early Intervention: An Ethical Perspective" (1986). The Turnbulls used the words of adults with disabilities to argue for the importance of "valuing and loving the totality of the child," solidifying a sense of intactness that includes facilitating self-image and self-esteem.

Historically it appears that this dehumanizing stance toward children often spreads to their families, resulting in a distancing, manifested by an emphasis on deficit and pathology in the family system. A more empathetic approach was underutilized.

HISTORY OF THROUGH THE LOOKING GLASS

Before establishing Through the Looking Glass, from 1974 its founding staff worked with families with adolescents or adults with disabilities at the Berkeley Center for Independent Living. The independent living program context meant that family support and intervention were frequently provided during the transition from nursing homes or parental homes to independent living. Intervention also emphasized maintaining independent living and family functioning, for instance, after the exacerbation of a disability or after traumatic injury. Through the Looking Glass was founded as a separate agency in 1982, focusing on earlier preventive family intervention in situations where there was disability in an infant, child, or parent.

The agency was founded with two primary missions:

1. to create, demonstrate and encourage resources and model early intervention services which are nonpathological and empowering, and which integrate the perspectives of adults or parents with disabilities as well as parents of children with disabilities;
2. to emphasize a life-cycle perspective, so that services to babies with disabilities and their families are informed with awareness of issues and possibilities for adults with disabilities. Services to parents with disabilities are informed by awareness of the implications of issues in the parent's family of origin and history.

To implement these missions the agency has from the outset been staffed primarily by professionals with personal disability experience. These "peer professionals" represent diverse family perspectives: e.g., people with disabilities, adult children of people with disabilities, spouses, parents, or siblings. Clinical work and research has bridged the parenting life cycle by focusing on families where there is an infant with a disability as well as families where there is a parent with a disability. Clinical training of people with personal disability experience has been a long-term goal and practice.

In 1982 the agency initiated services by mental health professionals who were "peers" with the participants. This occurred at a time when this was not acceptable practice in the Bay Area. It was the first infant mental health program in the country to focus on disability issues, and apparently the first to blend family therapy with infant mental health approaches.

From early on the agency offered support groups facilitated by "peer professionals" for parents of babies or young children with disabilities as well as for parents with disabilities. Home visits were part of the intervention strategy. Here peer professionals utilized a blend of infant mental health and family therapy approaches in working with disability issues. Implementing projects described below, staffing gradually expanded to 15 by 1993, including psychologists, social workers, marriage, child and family therapists, infant educators, childbirth educators, occupational therapists, rehabilitation engineers, and researchers. Professionals without personal disability experience, or "nonpeers," were integrated into the staff, thus helping to enhance its cultural diversity. All disability categories, such as cognitive, physical and sensory disability, are included in the clientele and research participants, and approximately half are families of color, from varied cultures. A full spectrum of families is involved with the agency, with diversity in functioning and stress level as well as ethnicity and socioeconomic status.

In 1984 an interviewing project with parents who had sensory or physical disabilities and an analysis of the literature resulted in a chapter on pregnancy and birthing by persons with disabilities (M. Kirshbaum and G. Rinne). Many of the interviewed parents with disabilities, a particularly articulate and independent group, reported that it was common for professionals to question their ability to care for their babies. Implied was questioning parents' awareness of the babycare implications of their own disabilities. For instance, a deaf parent would be asked, "but how will you hear your baby cry?"! Such questioning was often viewed as offensive and undermining of self-esteem at a time of high stress and vulnerability at the outset of parenthood. Unfamiliar with how adults with disabilities lived independently in the community, some professionals found it hard to envision the situation of a supposedly dependent person with a disability caring for a dependent baby.

The literature search for the chapter revealed a remarkable scarcity of good quality research material. From the point of view of the disability community, existing research was often attitudinally negative and pathological in emphasis and in the language or hypotheses chosen. Assumptions tended to be made about analogies between mental illness and physical disability without significant familiarity or knowledge of the latter. Speculations, however interesting, were not grounded in clinical or fieldwork expertise with adults with physical disabilities. Practical material for service providers and parents was also scarce.

The interviewing project and clinical work also revealed that parents with disabilities felt isolated and deprived of role models. At this time, in the early 1980s, there were remarkably few images of parents with disabilities in the media, so that children with disabilities had matured without experiencing such images.

In response to all these issues we decided to conduct research that included videotaped documentation of baby care by people with physical disabilities. In 1985 the Easter Seal Research Foundation funded a 3-year groundbreaking research project on the interaction between mothers with physical disabilities and their babies. Basic care in 11 families was regularly videotaped from birth through toddlerhood, and there was an analysis of how babies and parents reciprocally dealt with disability obstacles during this care. Disabilities included different degrees of spinal cord injury and cerebral palsy, as well as spina bifida, multiple sclerosis, and postpolio. Early adaptation in infants, as early as one month of age, and ingenuity and inventiveness in parents were documented, despite the absence of community resources or specialized parenting equipment. The project is described in more detail in "Parents with Physical Disabilities and their Babies" (M. Kirshbaum, 1988).

This publication led to hundreds of requests for information. Consequently, we established Through the Looking Glass' national newsletter, entitled "Parenting with a Disability." The result is a database of now more than 700 individuals or groups in the U.S. and abroad. The longitudinal videotapes from this and subsequent research projects have primarily been used to stimulate parents' problem-solving process and to educate and sensitize professionals in numerous fields. Since the founding of the agency more than 4000 diverse professionals have received training regarding parents with disabilities and other family disability issues. Presentations have dealt with a wide range of topics, such as pregnancy and birthing by people with disabilities, intervention in families with progressive disabilities, the formation of the infant/parent relationship when a baby has a disability, and issues in therapy by people with personal disability experience. Training material and videotape excerpts have been used by the national media, providing an opportunity to impact broader attitudinal change. Research results have also informed court proceedings, as well as the development of legislation and public policy, regarding parents with disabilities.

The National Institute of Disability and Rehabilitation Research (NIDRR), U.S. Department of Education, has been particularly supportive of the development of Through the Looking Glass' work. They awarded the agency three consecutive "Innovative" grants (1986-89) for research and demonstration projects concerning:

1. the effectiveness of clinical services offered to disabled baby or disabled parent families by "peer professionals" with personal disability experience;
2. the effectiveness of professional training regarding families with parents or babies with disabilities, when offered by "peer-professionals";
3. the bridging of the two populations of parents with disabilities and parents of babies with disabilities in an effort to provide a sense of future possibilities to the parents of the babies. In addition, previously completed videotapes were used in order to stimulate the problem-solving process for new parents with disabilities.

Clinical experience during these projects surfaced other critical issues that needed to be addressed. Through the Looking Glass had dealt with a number of cases where removal of disabled parents' babies had occurred, or was a strong possibility. Assessment of the functioning of these parents did not, prior to Through the Looking Glass involvement, include provision or recognition of the need for adaptive parenting equipment or the teaching of adaptive techniques. The involved professionals were not aware that such provision would be crucial to a fair assessment of parenting capability or the infant/parent relationship. To deal with the disability factors influencing the infant/parent relationship, Through the Looking

Glass staff took on the task of providing parenting equipment and techniques. The immediate dilemma was the absence of such equipment on the market, with a few customized solutions referred to in publications, and an absence of funding for the development of such equipment for low income families. Again, funding was sought to address these important issues.

As a result, Through the Looking Glass currently has a 3-year (1991-94) Field-Initiated Research grant from NIDRR for the purpose of "Developing Adaptive Equipment and Techniques for Physically Disabled Parents and their Babies Within the Context of Psychosocial Services (#H133G10146)." This project builds upon the previously videotaped documentation of problem-solving in parents with disabilities. This store of creative solutions is combined with technological expertise and family support via infant mental health services.

A core concept is the utilization of the expertise of parents with disabilities and their family members. A unique collaboration integrates parent or peer expertise with technology or biomechanics, infant mental health and family intervention services. The demonstrated services are intended to maximize the functioning of a broad spectrum of families where there are parents with physical disabilities and babies. It is hoped that the project will alleviate stress in the families, and sometimes even prevent the removal of infants from their parents. One of the products, available in 1994, will be "Guidelines for Assessment and Intervention." This document will inform child protective services and parenting professionals regarding services and assessment of parental capability which are sensitive and appropriate to disability. A Resource Catalogue will also be published. This will include: (1) photographs, illustrations and design information regarding the adaptive parenting equipment we have developed, existing equipment we have modified, and available usable existing equipment we have found on the market; (2) national and international resources for parents with disabilities; and (3) an extensive bibliography of this subject.

While serving parents with physical disabilities, we discovered that in our region there was a shocking lack of services to parents considered to be developmentally disabled. We were receiving referrals for such families from child protective services, subsequent to abuse and neglect incidents. By that time multifaceted damage to children and families had already occurred. After many years of advocacy, in 1990 a large preventive intervention project received funding from the system serving people with developmental disabilities, the California State Department of Developmental Services. This project focuses on serving individuals labelled as being mentally retarded or as dual diagnosis (MR and psychiatric) during pregnancy and parenting. During pregnancy each family is served by a childbirth educator and an infant mental health clinician. These services focus on enhancing understanding of the birthing process, self-care, preparation for newborn care and parenthood, stabilizing the home environment, and labor coaching. After birth each family has an infant development specialist and the same infant mental health clinician. At this point the workers provide ongoing assessment and facilitation of the baby's development, teach parenting skills, support parent/infant attachment and interaction, and address couple/family issues. After the child is three the developmental services end while the other services continue. All services are provided through regular home visits, twice or more per week.

Through the Looking Glass has just been awarded funding by NIDRR for a National Rehabilitation Research and Training Center for Families of Adults with Disabilities (PR Award # H133B30076) from 1993-97, which will include numerous research and training projects encompassing the production of training modules and the establishment of a national clearinghouse.

THEORETICAL FRAMEWORK

Core criteria underlying choices in research focus are utility to families and service providers and the potential for social change. For instance, videotaping is frequently done in research, partly because it provides images and material useful for clinical intervention as well as for practitioner training, behavioral or social change via the media.

From the outset, Through the Looking Glass has emphasized a nonpathological model, maintaining that the paradigm vitiating the work of professionals in the disability field is the social pathology or medical model, focusing on the deficits or "deviance" of people with disabilities and their families. An alternative paradigm suggested considers personal and social context, an ethnographic or systems perspective, and an emphasis on studying and facilitating strengths in families with disabilities.

Through the years nonpathological models regarding disability have become more common. Like ours, they frequently are consumer-driven. Such models have tended to focus on positive situations or issues to such an extent that they sometimes seem weakened in their relevance to a broad spectrum of families and practitioners. For instance, in laudable efforts to empower parents, systems may be constructed which omit consideration of the service needs of parents who are involved with children's protective services or parents with psychiatric disabilities.

Our own conceptual model has been tested through experience with many families who have multiple stressors even without considering disability. Through extensive examination of the literature, training of professionals, interagency work and court testimony we have learned that it is crucial to directly confront pathological assumptions and attitudinal biases impacting families with disability. Our conceptual approach has therefore evolved into a depathologizing model. For instance, the new Research and Training Center will have a research project that confronts issues that are likely to be sensitive and controversial in the disability community–e.g., the degree to which babies are stressed while adapting to their parents' disability needs, behavior management and parentification in families where there are parents with physical disability. These issues are tackled because we have found them to be recurring concerns of many mental health professionals and parents. However, we attempt to depathologize the "negative" issues by, in the same study, identifying aspects of the relationships between parents with disabilities and their children which lead to positive child outcomes.

Another example of grappling with pathology began in the early years of Through the Looking Glass when professionals questioned the ability of parents with disabilities to physically care for their babies. We chose a study investigating the nature of this care. When we analyzed how many extremely resourceful parents with disabilities elicited cooperation in their children without overburdening

them, this information guided intervention with famil
more stressed and less resourceful.

Through our willingness to become involved wi
challenging family situations and public policy issu
has evolved where our evaluation and intervention are sought by
parents and systems advocating for parents, as well as systems
advocating for children. In the midst of these, often legal, conflicts,
we attempt to maintain a balanced depathologizing and relation-
ship-oriented focus.

Case anecdotes will illustrate how, in our clinical work, we use a
family systems approach and an infant mental health emphasis on
observation of the infant/parent relationship to discern first what is
adaptable, understandable and even common given disability experience, rather than leaping to pathological interpretations.

CLINICAL ANECDOTES

Teamwork, between two parents with disabilities or a parent with
a disability and a parent or attendant who is able-bodied, is commonly documented by our videotape research. Being familiar with
adaptive teamwork patterns informs the assessment of couple difficulties with achieving this collaboration and informs the choice of
appropriate interventions. For instance, a Filipino/Japanese couple
was referred to us with a failure-to-thrive, extremely irritable one-
month premature baby. The father was gradually becoming blind,
and a general behavioral pattern was emerging: overfunctioning by
the sighted wife and underfunctioning by the visually disabled husband. The wife believed that her husband was completely incapable
of caring for the baby. This was reinforced by cultural attitudes
toward disability. The result was enormous couple conflict, in particular, arguing and shouting at one another while caring for this
extremely sensitive baby. Due to the sighted mother's tension and
fastidiousness the diapering was extremely prolonged, and the baby
was regularly building up to a peak of crying that was exhausting
and alarming. One of the earliest interventions with this family was
to get the couple to channel their disputes into times when they
weren't handing their baby, framed as to help his digestion. During
the sessions the therapists, instead, experimented with the couple

working as a team, e.g., the father soothing and containing the baby with his hand on the baby's chest and arms while the mother diapered. Thus, the changes were less prolonged and stressful for the baby, and the experience of helping their baby together was seeded. This is only a fragment illustrating a concrete intervention combining infant mental health and family therapy approaches during diapering. It occurred within the context of long-term therapeutic work dealing with a history of cumulative losses, cultural differences between the parents, teaching parenting adaptations regarding blindness, and other major issues.

An infant mental health approach helps one understand how a traumatic history impacts interaction between a parent and a baby. One also needs to understand how disability may complicate the trauma and the relationship. A parent labelled with retardation had just moved from a supervised residential setting into independent living. She was leaving her mobile baby in a highchair for long hours as she labored to make the new apartment spotlessly clean. Questioning this behavior directly or literally was fruitless. The meaning of the behavior had to be elicited. She had a history of removal of her four previous children by child protective services. Like many parents with cognitive disability, her understanding of the basis of the removal was very limited. She had focused on one concrete element in the removal–the allegation that her home had been messy. She was terrified that this baby too would be removed due to a messy house. Surfacing the meaning of the behavior it was then possible to help the mother–step by step and with repetition– clarify and reprocess this event. She gradually relaxed and allowed the baby mobility in the new setting.

We frequently have found mothers so intensely identified with their infants who have disabilities that these able-bodied mothers manifest disability symptoms. The clinicians working with such mothers have also cared for their own infants with disabilities and some have personally experienced such symptoms. The degree of our staff's personal and professional experience provides perspective so that one can assess the symptoms, without being unnecessarily alarming. Then, we can construct intervention that draws upon the "disability norm." A mother of a baby with truncated and weak arms was terrified when she began to experience weakness in her arms on awakening in the morning. The peer clinician was able to describe the analogous experiences of many other parents, normalizing, and reframing "the symptom" as "a way we seem to want to join with our babies, and hope to take away some of the disability, as if taking it on ourselves." In a more intense situation, when emergency surgery for a baby with a disability resulted in paralysis in an able-bodied mother, another peer clinician's crisis intervention was to more clearly join with the mother, citing her own experience of taking on her child's disability out of desperation to help. The "paralysis" quickly dissipated.

It is common for parents of children with disabilities to have undergone multiple traumatic events such as their babies' hospitalizations, surgeries, and medical emergencies. The impact of this cumulative trauma is frequently underestimated by professionals, and the parents may therefore be labelled as being overanxious, fixated in prolonged grieving, paranoid, or borderline, and this labeling may result in additional stress or underestimating of the potential for positive change. It is enlightening, rather, to apply the literature on post-traumatic stress, such as J.L. Herman's *Trauma and Recovery* (1992), to this population. Within a therapeutic relationship or a supportive parent group the sharing of pathologizing experiences with professionals can be part of a powerful "normalizing" and healing process.

Many parents feel traumatized by recurrent experiences which seem to dehumanize their babies with disabilities. This is a particular issue when disability stressors already strain one's ability to form an initial relationship with the baby (L. Milburn, personal communication, 1990). For instance, a parent may be having difficulty connecting to a baby with a disability, feeling alienated because of the personal and social connotation of disability. The baby may be unresponsive, irritable and/or unattractive, even repulsive, and may require a remarkable degree of vigilant care. The parent's grief and depression are another obstacle to forming a relationship. Overall the potential infant/parent relationship is in a tenuous and intensely vulnerable state. The usual difficulties in the couple transition to parenthood are intensified. At this point interventions and diagnostic explorations in the medical realm may feel like an assault on these shaky relationships.

One example was a dysmorphology evaluation, a medical examination that attempted to discern whether a baby had a syndrome, or a number of anomalies that have been recognized as occurring together, due to heredity or mutation. A team of physicians examined the baby's and parents' physical characteristics. Then a written report was sent to the parents, listing the baby's relevant body parts and the extent to which they were normal or abnormal. To the parents these authorities seem to have viewed their baby, not as a person to be loved, but as a thing. He had been dissected—a sum of his parts. For weeks the mother would be nursing her baby and suddenly shift to "their view," seeing his finger as malformed or watching for a change in the shape of his neck which would further substantiate a syndrome implying retardation.

While pursuing more sensitive medical intervention through professional training, a Through the Looking Glass clinician gave the parents an empathetic setting for discharging their anger at the perceived medical assault. She also facilitated their perception of the baby as a little person and unique individual. Later, when they felt it necessary to undergo a follow-up diagnostic session with a team of dysmorphologists, the clinician had the parents study and take notes on the behavior of the physicians and write these up in a statement that would contribute to physician sensitivity training by peer professionals. They weathered the appointment well and reported the dysmorphologist behavior with humor and insight. The intervention was intended to reverse the usual pattern of doctor/patient interaction in such situations. The power and observer status of the parents was enhanced with their analysis respectfully channeled into positive social change. Their expertise would be used to ameliorate the deficits of physicians. A grim experience had been infused with a certain mischievousness and humor. All this served as an antidote to their original traumatizing experience.

The work with babies who have disabilities and their families informs the work with parents with disabilities and their families. For instance, we attend to the old memories of early trauma surrounding the birth of a disabled infant that typically resurfaces in grandmothers when their disabled adult child gives birth. A generation later we start to address that lingering and retriggered pain as it complicates the family support for the adult-disabled child who is now a parent. In one family this took the form of intense mother/ daughter conflict during the pregnancy of a young woman with moderate cerebral palsy. The parental family had tolerated their daughter's independent living, working, and forming a sexual relationship. The mother was having great difficulty tolerating the idea of her daughter bearing a child and was pressuring for abortion, insisting that she would be unable to physically care for a child. The expectant mother sought counseling and adaptive parenting information and on this basis decided to continue the pregnancy. She began attending a support group for parents with disabilities. Sessions with a clinician who was also the parent of a child with a disability provided the grandmother with the first "peer counseling" regarding her relationship with her daughter. An occupational therapist, herself a mother with a disability, showed the mother and daughter videotapes of parents with comparable disabilities caring for their babies, and started discussing ideas about adaptive parenting equipment that we could develop. After the birth the new mother gradually proved her abilities and asserted herself regarding excessive help from the grandmother. A subsequent birth was calmly accepted and both children are thriving.

The work with parents who have disabilities also informs the work with parents and their babies with disabilities. A Chinese-American mother felt intense shame about having had a baby with a physical disability. Distraught and withdrawn she would only accept services from another parent. In the course of providing intervention with this family the clinician mentioned our work with parents who have disabilities. Many months later, when the mother was ready, she elicited information about how disabled adults live. She would have liked to ask them directly but wouldn't intrude. Told about our videotapes of adults with disabilities taking care of their children she requested a viewing. The tapes had great impact on her and her husband. Charged material surfaced regarding their original difference in attitude regarding the survival of their baby and underlying contrasts in their attitude about disability in general. Airing and assimilating their own differences made a difference in their son becoming less intolerable. Parental problem-solving in the tapes then provided an impetus for the father to begin inventing attractive adaptive play equipment for his child, pulling him more centrally into parental involvement. The tapes seeded the first shared hope for a future and a full life for their son. The parents began to participate together in community programs dealing with creative adaptive solutions regarding disability in children.

Our research has documented how the adaptive collaboration between the parent with a disability and the baby develops gradually over time, apparently beginning during the first weeks of life. Removal into foster care may disrupt this adaptive process, obfuscating the potential of the dyad. In one assessment situation, after a long-term out-of-home placement, a toddler had an avoidant and aversive reaction to his severely disabled mother. A psychologist with limited disability experience was interpreting this aversion as the baby's response to the parent's intrapsychic pathology. The Through the Looking Glass clinician had noted the child's auditory sensitivity and wondered if he could be frightened of the parent's motorized wheelchair. She began experimenting with having people with whom he was comfortable sit with him in the wheelchair. This made the toddler upset and anxious. She then tried having the mother play with the child out of her wheelchair on the floor. During the first of these "floor" visits he played with his mother for the first time. By the second such visit his previous pervasive anxiety had seemingly disappeared and he initiated vocalizing, social play and "en face" positioning with her. These had all been absent before. By the third such visit he was willing for the first time to be fed and touched by the mother, laughed with her and started playing with the footrest of her wheelchair. This compelling work would have needed to continue, consolidating the relationship to the "floor mom," while simultaneously desensitizing the child to the wheelchair, then working on the relationship to the "mom in wheelchair." Only at that point could you have assessed the potential of the parent/baby relationship.

We have been drawn into poignant and tragic situations where ignorance about disability has irreparably damaged an already tenuous chance for parent/child reunification. The department of social services involved us with a family after the baby, who was removed at birth, was already six months old. The newborn infant had a positive tox screen, indicating maternal substance abuse during the pregnancy. This teenage African-American mother lived in a particularly hazardous Oakland housing project with her alcoholic and abusive mother. She had been given drugs by family and friends who served as attendants. She had quadriplegia from spinal cord injury, and was said to be uncooperative with substance abuse treatment. However, she had only been referred to two different programs which were inaccessible to her wheelchair and refused to deal with her catheter in order to do urine analyses. She had been instructed to travel to these programs on the bus, though bus wheelchair access in her town is largely mythical. The social worker had been unaware of disability transportation systems or the few disability sensitive substance abuse programs. She described the mother as forming no relationship to her baby during the weekly visitations. Since the baby had been born the mother had been provided no assistance in order to make it possible for her to hold or care for her baby in any way. As a result the able-bodied grandmother did the care or left the baby in a playpen during the visits. During the first visit the Through the Looking Glass clinician saw a depressed mother who indeed appeared estranged from and disinterested in her baby. This visit focused on viewing videotapes of parents with disabilities, as requested by the mother. At the end of the visit she asked for assistance in holding and feeding her baby. In the second visit, with the use of simple pillows and frontpacks the mother was able to hold and feed her baby for the first time since her birth. She tenderly nuzzled and murmured to her baby, caressing, as one greets a baby immediately after birthing.

In contrast, a mother with an equally severe disability has been receiving services from Through the Looking Glass since her premature baby was sent home from neonatal intensive care. During home visits we have developed the adaptive parenting equipment she has needed to provide totally independent care of her baby. A babycare tray attached to her motorized wheelchair kept the vulnerable baby close and minimized the stress of positional changes. Later an elevated play area at wheelchair level allowed the child to be mobile and available for play with the mother. Adaptations to crib, highchair, bottles, diapers, changing table, toys, and safety gates maximized the capability of the mother. Technology provision and adaptive problem-solving by an occupational therapist has been offered in addition to infant mental health services, both provided through home visits. Despite the high risk childhood history, in out-of-home placement of this mother, the relationship between parent and child continues to flourish.

The blending of technology and family intervention can be complex. We are constantly grappling with the clinical implications of this blend. Providing adaptive equipment and techniques can produce quick change that is difficult for families to assimilate. For instance, a Samoan mother with hemiplegia gave birth to her first child. She ordinarily walked with a cane, but had balance problems and use of only one arm. A pattern of underfunctioning by the mother and the stress of the transition to parenthood seemed to trigger anger and physical abuse in the father. A prompt attempt was made to maximize the mother's physical ability to function by providing an adapted crib and a reclined stroller with good support so the mother could move the baby from room to room safely. It was hoped that the ability to do her own baby care would eliminate one element of the need to remain in a battering relationship. Yet the requested equipment tended not to be used. The clinician, a woman with a disability, had to backtrack and focus on intervention that confronted the abuse and supported a tolerance of a change in the balance of functioning in the couple. The abuse did not reoccur and there was subsequently a very gradual increase in the disabled woman's functioning, proudly reported, over many years. She was much more active in the care of her next two children, and her husband increasingly took pride in her accomplishments and her strength.

A family requested adaptive parenting equipment for the care of their second child. They felt that the lack of early baby care by the disabled father undermined the relationship between the father and the first child. While developing the equipment for this baby's care, we also provided therapy to address the relationship with the first child. Otherwise, we can predict that the enhancement of the relationship with the second child would intensify problems with the first, creating additional stress in the family.

CONCLUSIONS

Expertise regarding disability, or familiarity with the disability "norm," serves the depathologizing process. Awareness of disability issues throughout the life cycle further enriches intervention.

In evaluating capability and intervening to enhance it in a parent or a family, disability expertise can make it possible to sort out disability issues and obstacles from psychosocial ones. For instance, if one makes it possible for a severely disabled parent to adaptively give care and relate to her baby, providing support and resources for the family unit, then one can evaluate whether the parent is motivated and psychologically able at this point to maintain an appropriate relationship with a child. One can expect a sudden increase in parental functioning to be stressful. However, one can consider whether the relationship begins to develop at this point, or, instead, the parent becomes threatened by the reality of this possibility and opts out of the situation; for instance, by retreating into substance abuse or relinquishing custody. Addressing disability issues appropriately brings clarity to the situation.

At Through the Looking Glass we approach disability work primarily from within disability culture(s), by emphasizing service delivery by clinicians with personal disability experience. The initial advantage of such staffing is the escalation of the process of forming therapeutic relationships. Other advantages include the provision of role models, the naturalness of empathetic and non-pathological approaches, and the available expertise regarding disability. The disadvantages include the precipitousness of the development of trust. Clients frequently need to be slowed in their outpouring of material so there is time for a solid sustaining relationship to develop beyond the initial identification. Therapists need careful supervision and consultation to manage countertransference issues and utilize the full potential of their peer status. Increasingly we have integrated non-peers into our staff, who are doing what is essentially cross-cultural therapy and enriching the dialogue in the organization. Rather than encourage mental health services that segregate disability and emphasize "taking care of our own," we would like to encourage the development of staffing that is strengthened by both peer and non-peer perspectives. Through the Looking Glass has found that its "melting pot" of diverse viewpoints has been a fertile source of creativity in clinical intervention as well as in the development of service delivery models and the encouragement of social change.

The cross-cultural notion and the characterization of disability as cultural in nature is a function partly of the intensity of the psychological experience, and so much of this intensity has been the result of social stigma and obstacles and nontherapeutic intervention. One can only speculate about the eventual impact of integration, assimilation and social change on the cultural status and psychological experience of disability. At this point, during intervention a great deal of pain is still caused because of pathologizing. This form of distancing from families is still a particular problem in the mental health field. The family therapy specialty has the potential for a less pathological and more systems-oriented approach, yet few family therapists have chosen to work with disability issues. It is paradoxical that disability is still considered as alien, even unspeakable, when it is actually so remarkably commonplace in families. To relate to clients with disability issues, therapists without such experience can draw upon their insight concerning resilience in the face of reactive responses to loss, trauma, and social oppression. As a clinician working with our families, in essence, you will need to discern and respect difference, but also to allow empathy and recognition of commonality, providing what you may well want for your own family someday.

REFERENCES

Herman, J. L. (1992). *Trauma and Recovery.* New York: Basic Books.

Kirshbaum, M. (1988). Parents with physical disabilities and their babies. *Zero to Three, 8*(5), 8-15.

Kirshbaum, M., & Rinne, G. (1985). The disabled parent. In M. Auvenshine & M. Enriquez (Ed.), *Maternity Nursing: Dimensions of Change* (pp. 645-669). Belmont, CA: Wadsworth Inc.

Turnbull, A. P. & Turnbull, H. R. (1986). Stepping back from early intervention: An ethnical perspective. *Journal of the Division for Early Childhood, 10,* 106-117.

Serving Holocaust Survivors and Survivor Families

Zev Harel

SUMMARY. This article reviews and discusses the characteristics and needs of aging survivors of the Holocaust. Journalistic and historic accounts have documented the gruesome details of the Holocaust and, to a lesser extent, the consequences of these harrowing experiences. Professional and scientific efforts in the immediate postwar years have aimed to specify and understand the mental health consequences of the Holocaust in survivors. Efforts have also been directed to aid their adjustment to the postwar years.

The article addresses attitudinal and assumptional issues first. These include assumptions and generalizations prevalent in the literature concerning the effects of the Holocaust on survivors. Second, conceptual issues are explored in order to facilitate a better understanding of the nature and needs of victims of the Holocaust. These include a review of mental health consequences of extreme stress, the role and importance of coping style and coping resources, and the interaction of stress, aging and resources in later years of life. Next, this article offers directions for professional efforts aimed at aiding the adjustment to aging of Holocaust survivors and members of their families.

INTRODUCTION

Research indicates that survivors remember frequently the horrors of their past and continue to cope, to this day, with the memories of

Zev Harel is Professor of Social Work, Cleveland State University, Cleveland, OH.

[Haworth co-indexing entry note]: "Serving Holocaust Survivors and Survivor Families." Harel, Zev. Co-published simultaneously in *Marriage & Family Review* (The Haworth Press, Inc.) Vol. 21, No. 1/2, 1995, pp. 29-49; and: *Exemplary Social Intervention Programs for Members and Their Families* (ed: David Guttmann, and Marvin B. Sussman) The Haworth Press, Inc., 1995, pp. 29-49. Multiple copies of this article/chapter may be purchased from The Haworth Document Delivery Center [1-800-3-HAWORTH; 9:00 a.m. - 5:00 p.m. (EST)].

their adverse experiences along with the new challenges of aging. While some survivors demonstrated strength and resiliency in overcoming numerous adversities, others were severely traumatized and severely scarred. Still others recouped inner resources and relied on environmental resources to go on and lead productive lives.

For many survivors, despite the memories of their observed and/or experienced acts of persecution, advanced years of life are a period of growth and contentment, experienced in a variety of ways. Many survivors use these later years to embark on new life styles which include intellectual, social and recreational pursuits. Others engage in volunteer and other altruistic endeavors. They may engage in extensive travel, spend time in warmer climates, and participate in civic activities. These survivors are likely to live lives similar to those enjoyed by "well aged."

There are also survivors, however, for whom adjustment and adaptation to the challenges of later years may be difficult. A decline in health and functional status may lead to the necessity to disengage involuntarily from various activities and social relationships. Furthermore, losses associated with aging, including reduced income and financial resources, death of a significant family member or friend, severe disability or deterioration may activate vulnerabilities related to past traumatic experiences.

Later years are characterized by a need to integrate and come to terms with past experiences. For many survivors, this challenge is especially difficult because of the wish to forget along with the need to remember and bear witness. On the one hand they have easy recollections and intrusive imageries of the past while, on the other hand, they have considerable difficulty coming to terms with such memories.

The primary purpose of this article is to review and discuss scientific and professional perspectives on mental health consequences of stress and extreme stress and discuss possible directions for aiding the adjustment of aging survivors of the Holocaust. Practice efforts of health and human service professionals need to be guided, in the author's view, by one or more of the following objectives: (a) provide older individuals and families with effective services that are efficiently delivered, (b) allow older persons as much discretion as possible over the services they use, (c) encourage and support family members and friends in caring for older persons, and (d) enhance the coping resources of older persons and members of their informal caregivers (Harel et al., 1985). These objectives are important in work with all aged; these are also applicable in work with people who endured traumatic stresses in their lives and, when applied, are likely to lead to more effective services.

In the fields of health and human services, assumptions made about the nature and needs of the clientele determine, to a considerable extent, the desired practice objectives and the techniques employed in professional services. Historically, beliefs held by professionals about the nature and needs of individuals and groups have determined treatment strategies and care practices (Harel et al., 1984). For this reason, the exploration of perceptions held about the Holocaust and about survivors by members of various professional groups as well as those held by survivors themselves is important. A better understanding of Holocaust survivors by professionals is likely to enhance their ability to serve their needs and represent their interests.

Similarities in perceptions are likely to facilitate meaningful communications between survivors and members of professional groups. Contradictory perceptions and/or misguided assumptions about the nature and needs of individuals and families seeking professional help are likely to lead to mistrust and alienation and hinder the fostering of necessary professional relationships and, in turn, impede the delivery of effective services. Survivors seeking professional help need the assurance of professional sensitivity and understanding to their concerns and needs if they are to benefit from help in times of need. Survivors' perceptions that the professional community is understanding and respectful of their sufferings, losses and painful memories should enhance the ability of professionals to serve their needs. Therefore, the review and discussion of the literature on the mental health implications of extreme stress on survivors held by professionals is indeed necessary.

THE HOLOCAUST LITERATURE

The Holocaust literature, in the aftermath of World War II, generated a general conclusion that survivors, as a consequence of their traumatic experiences, have suffered lasting physical, mental, psychological, and social impairments, including severe handicaps in their personal and social functioning. The literature indicates that not only have survivors themselves been impacted by their traumatic experiences, but that also their children are likely to have experienced psychological and social effects that are directly related to the experiences of their survivor parents (Chodoff, 1963; Krystal, 1968).

A review of the clinical literature dealing with the effects of the Holocaust on survivors continues to reveal an overwhelming pathological emphasis (Steinberg, 1989)–an emphasis which, from the comfortable perspective afforded by hindsight, appears to have been regrettable. In addition to the scientifically questionable generalizations, earlier conclusions about the effects of the Holocaust may have added a serious burden on survivors and children of survivors. This burden is being reflected in the fact that survivors and children of survivors were labeled as "damaged," being emotionally and socially impaired.

Survivors were characterized as suffering from various configurations of symptoms, identified in these writings as the "typical concentration camp syndrome," a label which implied serious impairment in psychological and social well-being (Chodoff, 1963). Survivors were also characterized by "survival guilt," consisting of feelings of guilt brought about by feelings that they had survived the Holocaust, while their relatives and friends have been killed (Chodoff, 1963). In addition, one of the writers asserted that Jews, as a consequence of 1,500 years of degradation learned to accept and internalized their enemies' views about themselves which led to feelings that they actually deserved to be punished and die (Krystal, 1968).

What strikes one as one reviews this literature from the sixties is the basic agreement among most of the writers to the conclusions that most, if not all, survivors have indeed suffered lasting physical, mental, psychological, and social impairments as a result of which they were severely handicapped in a variety of life situations. The following is a quote which may typify the characterization of Holocaust survivors as "damaged" in the clinical literature.

We've all been damaged, doctor, and I think we are all a bunch of rotten apples. We may look okay on the outside, but when you get to know us you will see that we are different and sick inside and no matter what happens our lives will never be normal again. (Oswald & Bittner, 1968, p. 1398)

Findings of more recent cross-sectional studies, including studies in which survivors and children of survivors were compared with appropriate comparison groups of similar sociocultural background who did not experience the Holocaust, suggest that earlier conclusions and generalizations based primarily on research conducted within the psychoanalytic tradition may have been overstated.

While there is evidence to indicate that a considerable number of survivors have been severely scarred by their experiences, there is also evidence that a large number of Holocaust survivors have adjusted well to their postwar experiences, and that they and their children enjoy reasonable states of psychological and social well-being (Harel et al., 1984; Kahana et al., 1988). The Holocaust literature that provided the bases for the conclusions that survivors suffered irreparable personal and social damage has serious theoretical and methodological limitations. There are two serious theoretical problems in the Holocaust literature from the sixties. Most of the studies draw exclusively on the psychoanalytic literature and almost completely neglect behavioral and social science perspectives. Most of the authors do not even indicate an awareness of this problem. The result is a serious gap in the informational and analytical content of these studies. Second, attempts have been made in many of these writings to draw broader theoretical inferences and generalizations from their observations and/or research than what their data justified (Harel et al., 1984; Steinberg, 1989).

Several authors have questioned the utility and wisdom of applying psychoanalytic models and the excessive reliance on unconscious processes for the explanation of the effects that the Holocaust experience had on survivors (DesPres, 1976). The psychoanalytic literature does not take into consideration the objective realities of the environmental situation in the concentration camps and the environmental conditions and social conditions in which Holocaust survivors lived in subsequent years (Harel et al., 1984).

Early studies on the effects of the Holocaust on survivors have methodological shortcomings as well. Most studies have employed small and nonrepresentative samples drawn in most instances from occasionally available captive and nonrepresentative groups. Virtually all of the cited reports are based on observations of nonrandom samples, either those seeking help or those applying for restitution and thus, inclined to emphasize not only the atrocities inflicted upon them but also the perceived subsequent consequences. Finally, while generalizing about the entire survivor population, most investigators employed no other groups to compare the survivors studied.

In recent years, a number of studies in which behavioral science perspectives have been applied to the study of long-range effects of the concentration camp experiences on survivors concluded that, contrary to the conclusions derived during the sixties, there were no concentration camp syndromes identifiable in the majority of survivors and that consequences of incarceration and concentration camp experiences may be manifested in a number of different ways. These studies concluded that survivors, while scarred by their experiences, and thinking frequently about their losses and experiences during the Holocaust, have made remarkable recoveries and adjustments. Authors question the notion of survivor guilt, the presence of emotional blunting in survivors, and the extremely maladaptive psychological influence of parents' experiences on children of survivors (Harel, 1984; Klein-Parker, 1988).

These more recent studies raised serious questions about earlier conclusions and generalizations based primarily on research conducted within the psychoanalytic tradition. Psychoanalytic perspectives do not take into consideration findings which indicate that the effects of stress on individuals vary because they are mediated through subjective psychological processes, which include both cognitive and emotional components. Furthermore, the effects of stress are mediated and moderated by various resources, including the personality structure of the individual and the social structure and the environmental condition into which he/she is embedded.

Behavioral science and social science perspectives provide a more useful perspective for the understanding of the long-range effects of the Holocaust on survivors. The stress literature provides a useful direction for the understanding of the Holocaust conditions and its aftermath. Survivors, during their war year experiences, had to focus their energies primarily, and almost exclusively, on survival. The situations they found themselves in posed constant threat to their lives. It is not surprising, therefore, that much of their energy, after the realization of the threats to their lives, was directed toward coping with the constant stresses in ways that would assure their survival.

Socio-environmental literature and research indicate that human behavior is affected to a very high degree by the objective environmental conditions, by the perception of the environmental demands and challenges, and by one's constant interaction with the environment (Germain, 1978; Gump, 1971).

Concentration camp conditions entailed situations where individuals had little or no ability to anticipate and predict outcomes on a day-to-day basis. While extensive states of physical degradation, deprivation, lack of food, extreme cold, and prolonged isolation were elements which characterized life in concentration camps and in prisoner of war camps, an additional important factor was the absence of conventional social structure. In concentration camps, conventional modes of behavior were rarely applicable, and the duration of the extreme situation and its complexity were, in most instances, unpredictable. Individuals in such circumstances were called upon to respond to conditions for which they were unprepared. At the same time, individuals in those situations were aware that failure to respond adequately held severe consequences for them, including the constant threat of death.

Holocaust survivors in the postwar years faced a triple challenge: first, they had to come to terms with and cope with their own traumatic experiences; second, they had to cope with the losses of family members and friends; and third, they were challenged to take on the demands associated with relocation to new environments. It is important to note that after an initial period of adjustment, the majority of Holocaust survivors took on the demands, challenges, and opportunities afforded them by their new environments and used effective coping strategies in their adjustment to conventional aspects of their postwar living conditions.

In their new environments, after liberation, they directed their energies toward establishing their personal identities and worked on assuring their socio-economic status, establishing social networks and social relations. They established themselves as family members, contributed to the formation and enhancement of Jewish communal life in the United States, Europe, and other parts of the world, and provided an important driving force in the establishment of the State of Israel and toward the assurance of its survival.

To assume that Holocaust survivors are a homogeneous group would obviously be inappropriate. While there is considerable evidence to indicate that some Holocaust survivors have been scarred to varying degrees by their experiences, there is also considerable evidence to indicate that a large fraction of the survivors not only adjusted well as individuals but also made substantial contributions to collective communal efforts in their new environments. While some survivors may be bothered by survivor guilt the majority among them suggest that those who committed the atrocities and those who stood by and did nothing are the ones who should feel guilty about their actions and/or inactions. Unfortunately, to date, there has been only limited scientific and professional effort directed towards the assessment of the strategies used by Holocaust survivors in coping with the long-range effects of the Holocaust and the factors that aided their adjustment in the postwar years. Today, the majority of survivors who are still alive are older persons, ranging in age from the high fifties to the nineties. The older among them are experiencing the health impairments and functional limitations associated with advanced age and are in need of health, long-term care, and supportive services. Some among them may also experience psychosocial problems and some of them may have difficulties with intrusive imageries and other mental health consequences of their traumatic wartime experiences.

MENTAL HEALTH CONSEQUENCES OF STRESS

Data from clinical observations and research suggest that stress may cause a wide range of physiological disorders, diseases, mental disorders, deviant behavior, and social pathology (Wilson et al., 1988). Individuals who endured extreme stress may experience immediately and in later years some degree of physical, social and psychological discomfort. Moreover, individuals who have endured extreme stress over a long period, may experience lasting physical and mental impairment. Extreme stress, frequently, has consequences on mental health. Systematic investigations indicate that it is not unusual for symptoms such as depression, startle responses, anxiety, hyperarousability, intrusive imagery and sleep disturbance, to persist for decades after the extreme stressful experience. Although stress research supports these conclusions, it also points to other lines of investigation.

Stress research indicates that there are substantial differences between individuals and groups in the way that they perceive and react to stressful situations and conditions (Lazarus et al., 1985). The effects of stress vary because they are mediated through subjective psychological processes which include both cognitive and emotional components, and because they are moderated by environmental, social and personal resources.

Although the specific mechanisms that cause post-traumatic difficulties in physiological functioning, mental health, and psychological adjustment are not well understood, it is clear that when extreme stressors are severe and enduring, behavioral, social, and psychological functioning may be potentially affected. However, reactions to extreme and traumatic stress vary significantly. Post-extreme stress adaptation and experiences, along with environmental and social resources, play a critical role in ameliorating extreme stress and enhancing well-being. Although factors such as social and emotional support, ego strength, and educational level moderate the effects of extreme stress, how these variables interact to determine different patterns of adjustment and psychological well-being during one's older age is unknown. The importance of moderating variables (i.e., environmental, personal and social resources available to the individual during and following the experience) in reducing the adverse consequences of the extreme stress response is just beginning to be understood.

There is also evidence which indicates that while the extreme stress experience may have intense negative effects, it may also generate some positive influences on the processes of continuity and change in the course of aging, most notably on the social system of the stress survivor (Elder & Clipp, 1988; Harel et al., 1984; Kahana et al., 1988; Steinitz, 1982). However, with the exception of few studies, little empirical evidence is available to substantiate definitive etiological explication. Furthermore, empirical analysis of the cumulative and interactive effects of these variables as they influence the mental health and adjustment to aging of extreme stress victims is largely absent, yet, in the literature.

COPING STYLES AND COPING STRATEGIES

There appears to be ample documentation for the importance that coping strategies have in dealing with critical life events and with extreme stressful conditions. Holocaust survivors, and other extreme stress victims, faced major challenges both during World War II and in the postwar years. During the Holocaust years they were challenged constantly, including by treats to their survival. In the postwar years they were faced with the need to come to terms with their observations and personal experiences and with losses of family members and friends. Second, they were challenged to resume life in environments which were neither understanding nor sympathetic to their experiences. Third, they were challenged to take on the demands and challenges of new environments and establish themselves as individuals, family members and members of new communities. To understand the coping styles and strategies of stress victims, it is essential, therefore, to address their historical experiences as well as the ways in which they cope with current demands and challenges, especially with their adjustment to aging (Shay, 1984).

The broad questions of coping, human adaptation or adjustment have been central to theoretical formulations dealing with personality, social behavior, and mental health. Social and behavioral scientists have long been interested in the human tendency to seek congruence (Germain, 1978) and in the ways that individuals cope with stress (Lazarus & Folkman, 1984).

In situations involving ordinary stresses or hassles of everyday life, one can anticipate that individual coping styles and strategies will largely explain variance in mental health. For survivors of extreme stress, however, less of the variance in outcomes may be a function of personal coping strategies.

The interactional dimensions of coping have been presented in the literature in the forms of coping as a mediator variable between specific situational stress and an outcome (Kahana et al., 1988), and as a transactional process involving an ongoing dynamic process (Lazarus & Folkman, 1984). In both of these approaches, coping is seen as dynamic responses to a specific environmental situation in an effort to reduce or avoid the effects of stress from that source.

Coping generally represents a response to a demand or challenge with an effort to reduce the extreme stress and reestablish a state of homeostasis. In the process of scientific and professional efforts to better understand the operational referents of coping, the variables of stress, coping and consequences of coping became gradually disentangled. Kahana, Harel and Kahana (1988) found empirically recurrent coping patterns among survivors distinguishing between instrumental, affective and avoidant strategies.

While there is general indication that adversity has detrimental consequences, there are also indications that individuals derive strength from adversity and may become better copers (Elder & Clipp, 1988; Kahana et al., 1988). Data indicate that initially effective copers remained effective copers over time, and that coping patterns were relatively stable over time (Eaton et al., 1982; Sigal et al., 1985).

A review of the literature on coping strategies suggests that strategies involving avoidant tactics may be effective in reducing pain, stress, and anxiety in some cases, whereas active strategies appear to be more effective in others (Suls & Fletcher, 1985). Research with Holocaust survivors indicated instrumental coping to be associated with psychological well-being, while escapist coping was associated with low psychological well-being (Kahana et al., 1988). However, data also indicate that stresses of aging in the form of reduced health, the onset of chronic illness, economic losses and social losses may present more difficult coping challenges for older survivors of extreme stress (Baider & Sarell, 1984; Wilson et al., 1988).

As survivors age, many among them have recurrent dreams and other intrusive imagery about their Holocaust experiences and their lost family members and friends. Some Holocaust survivors have returned to the sites where they experienced their personal horrors and also to the communities of origin and have shared their obıs and experiences with others. A significant number of st survivors have recorded their experiences in audio/video ı shared these with interested family members. Much of the research on coping is based on evidence from cross-sectional studies. Evidence concerning the effects of coping over time is awaiting empirical investigation employing longitudinal designs.

STRESS, AGING AND SOCIAL SUPPORT

Empirical evidence indicates that social support generally has a positive effect on the aged's functioning and psychological well-being (Harel & Deimling, 1984; Harel, 1988). Research shows that greater support received by the individual in the form of close relationships with family members, friends, acquaintances, co-workers, and the larger community decreases the likelihood that the individual will experience extreme stress or illness; thus, the level of well-being increases (Dean, 1986). There is also increasing evidence to indicate that greater social support is associated with better mental health among survivors of extreme stress (Elder & Clipp, 1988; Kahana et al., 1988; Wilson et al., 1988).

There is no clear indication as to why and how social support plays a role in preventing stress and illness. House (1981) suggests that social support may act as a buffer between stress and the individual's health. Dean (1986) concluded that social support may act either as an antecedent factor that reduces the effect of the undesirable experience or as a buffer following the experience.

The role that social interaction has in determining the mental health and well-being of the elderly is less clear. Previous research conducted by the author indicated that social interaction has a limited impact on the elderly's well-being. Social support and the perceived adequacy of social interaction were found to contribute more significantly to the elderly's mental health and well-being (Harel & Deimling, 1984; Harel, 1988; Larson, 1978).

Evidence is accumulating, however, concerning the buffering effect of social resources between stress and physical and mental health. Findings indicate that social networks exert a direct effect on reducing physical health symptoms. Social networks also act to reduce symptoms by buffering the effect of increased levels of stress. High levels of social support reduced the negative impact of stress on mental health. There are indications that specific types of social support (e.g., emotional support, integration, tangible help) buffer the impact of specific types of stressors (e.g., bereavement, crime, and social network crises). Furthermore, knowledge of social networks and social support were found to predict future health status with a high degree of certainty (Cohen & Wills, 1985; Krause, 1986). Older people who have more informational support and who provide support to others were found to report fewer symptoms of depression. Other studies indicate that life stress precipitates the onset of depression and that having a confidant can be protective in certain situations and that coping potency may be enhanced by social support. Mental health may also be enhanced by perceived availability of interpersonal resources that are responsive to the needs elicited by extreme stressful events (Ben-Sira, 1985; Cohen & Wills, 1985; Krause, 1987).

Evidence continues to accumulate indicating both direct and indirect effects of a nonsupportive social network on illness. The effects were not due to the amount of social contact or the quantity of social relationships, but to the extent to which a supportive network reduces feelings of isolation and provides support and help when needed. Stress resistant groups were found to have better family support than their counterparts in the distressed group (Dean, 1986; Holahan & Moos, 1985).

It is important to note that social networks cannot be viewed as inherently or consistently supportive. Social networks may be, in some instances, not only unsupportive but also damaging to older persons (Noelker & Harel, 1983). There is growing recognition to the burden created by the need to care for elder family members. Among spouse and daughter caregivers for impaired elders, cognitive incapacity was found to have a less important direct effect on caregiving extreme stress than disruptive behavior and impaired social functioning. The caregivers' perception of burden is often correlated with stress response and availability of social support (Jenkins et al., 1985). Another study suggests that there are two broad categories of factors that may have a bearing on the amount of stress that is created when an elderly parent comes to live with the host family. The first set pertains to social forces inherent in the relationship between the parent and the family, and the second relates to the health status of the parent. If the level of stress on family members is increased, without adding supports to help them cope with it, the likelihood of violence is increased, as a person and family can only handle so much (Galbraith & Davison, 1985). In the case of survivors of the Holocaust, the traumatic experience itself impacted in a major way on survivors' social resources; it resulted in loss of members of the family who comprised the essence of their earlier social networks.

The Holocaust literature of the sixties questioned the desire and ability of survivors to reconstruct new social networks through marriage, procreation and affiliation, the ability to establish meaningful and healthy social relationships with family members and friends and the ability to create friendships and to join formal and informal groups and organizations. Furthermore, it was generally accepted that the social interactions and social relations of survivors would be problematic as a consequence of their experiences during the Holocaust.

The comparison of Holocaust survivors and immigrants in the U.S. and Israel on social network, social interaction and social support in a recent cross-national cross-sectional study (Kahana et al., 1988; Harel et al., 1993) revealed that survivors had more stable families (lower divorce rates) and somewhat more extensive social network and slightly higher levels of social interaction.

Survivors were also more likely than members of the comparison groups to share with their children, family members, friends and co-workers everyday concerns and important concerns, including the discussion of sex issues and finances. Survivors were also somewhat more likely than members of the immigrant group to give and receive assistance with shopping, repairs, cooking, and finances and more likely to offer assistance in times of illness (Harel et al., 1993).

These findings indicate very clearly that in terms of social network, social interaction, self-disclosure and social support aging survivors of the Holocaust in the U.S. and Israel are doing as well and, in some instances, better than members of appropriate comparison groups.

The analyses of the importance of social network, social interaction, self-disclosure and social support for psychological well-being followed the general patterns found in the gerontological literature, indicating that those who have a caring social network and meaningful social interaction have slightly higher psychological well-being (Harel et al., 1993; Larson, 1978).

Indicators of social support revealed, again, what is typically found in the gerontological literature–namely receiving attention and assistance is associated with lower psychological well-being. Conversely, giving attention and assistance, and contributing to survivor and community social networks is more likely to be associated with better psychological well-being (Antonovsky, 1979; Harel et al., 1993).

In summary, it may be concluded that environmental, social, economic and personal resources have been consistently found to be associated with better mental and physical health in the aged. This association is also found in studies with survivors of extreme stress and in cross-sectional studies of Holocaust survivors. Social networks generally provide informal support to older individuals and families and, therefore, serve as a buffer between stress and physical and mental impairment. Conversely, losses in resources, and especially losses of irreplaceable social resources, serve as serious stressors in the lives of the aged. It is important to underscore, however, that social networks may also create stresses and this is especially evidenced in cases of heavy burdens of impaired aged.

AIDING THE ADJUSTMENT OF AGING SURVIVORS OF THE HOLOCAUST

Professional practice consists of: (a) attitudinal, ethical and value predispositions; (b) knowledge bases; and (c) practice skills. The purpose of this chapter is to address the first and second of these three components, namely to provide a better understanding of the ways in which older survivors of the Holocaust cope with their aging experiences, and to derive implications from the reviewed data for aiding professional practice efforts in the area of extreme stress. Sensitivity is a prerequisite in work with all aged and it is equally, if not more, important in practice with older persons coping with consequences of earlier extreme stress experiences.

Previous perspectives on the effects of the Holocaust have been based almost exclusively on generalizations derived from clinical studies anchored in the medical psychiatric tradition. More recent views on the long-range effects of extreme stress have begun to rely on findings from more systematic studies of stress and extreme stress which employed conceptual approaches anchored in the social and behavioral sciences. This chapter provides converging evidence from empirical studies concerning the effects of extreme stress, including the Holocaust on psychological well-being in late life. It substantiates the importance of post-stress factors for the mental health of aged coping with extreme stress consequences. More specifically, data from the reviewed studies suggest that adequate health, higher levels of economic resources and social resources, along with type of coping and personal resources are important determinants of mental health among all aged, including survivors of the Holocaust. It is important, therefore, that mental health professionals acquaint themselves with the empirical evidence from more recent research so as to better understand the experiences and service needs of older persons coping with extreme stress consequences.

There is a recognition in the professional literature that earlier practice assumptions based on the medical-psychiatric literature may have been limited in their utility to aid post-stress adjustment of survivors of extreme stress. Recent literature and research on mental health predictors among survivors of extreme stress, even though still limited, point to three major factors that are likely to affect the long term adaptation and well-being of aged extreme stress survivors. These include: (1) extreme stress factors (nature and duration of stress experiences); (2) current socio-demographic and socio-economic status and health; and (3) the current environmental, social and personal resources which effect modes of coping with conventional life and consequences of extreme stress experiences.

Findings of more recent research underscore the importance of recognizing that survivors of the Holocaust are not a homogeneous group and that their diversity provides important clues about the complex nature of post-traumatic adaptation. While there is considerable evidence to indicate that some survivors of the Holocaust have been scarred to varying degrees by their experiences, there is also considerable evidence to indicate that a large percentage of the survivors adjusted well as individuals and have become productive citizens in their new environments.

It is important to recognize that aging survivors of the Holocaust share many characteristics with older adults in the general population. Hence, conventional predictions of social and psychological well-being in late life (Larson, 1978) need to be considered. Findings indicate that mental health fifty years after the Holocaust is less affected by extreme stress experiences than the literature has indicated. However, the manner of coping with memories of the trauma and losses and the meaning found and attached to survivorship do play an important role in current mental health. The seminal work of Viktor Frankl (1969) provides evidence that coming to terms with survivorship and finding meaning in adversity and challenging life situations influence psychosocial well-being.

There is converging evidence in the gerontological literature regarding the universal importance of better health and functional status, adequate economic resources, and marriage for better psychological well-being in advanced years of life (Larson, 1978). There is also a clear indication in these data that coping style and the availability of social support and communication with members of one's primary group (i.e., spouse, children and other family members) and friends are indeed important contributors toward higher levels of psychological well-being and better mental health.

It is important to underscore, therefore, the following program and practice implications for work with older survivors of the Holocaust. There is a clear need for more programs that specifically address conditions within the older family unit and the needs of the unaffiliated older person. Programs which will enhance and strengthen the social network may be as clinically significant as implementing a medical procedure. There is a need for more adequate funding for supportive services in the community which may reduce care burdens. Service agencies should be able to develop and offer home health services, supportive equipment that enables greater self-care, and respite services.

It is important for health, mental health and social work practitioners to recognize that aging may generate constant stress in the lives of the elderly, one type of stress spilling over into other stresses over a long period of time. The subjective perception of the extreme stress and the perceived competence and resources needed to cope with the extreme stress may be at variance with their objective indications. These stresses are likely to interact with the consequences of earlier extreme stress experiences. There is a need to adequately assess the complexity of the current stress along with earlier stress experience complexity, along with the characteristics of family system and the social network and other resource features. Interventions need to be tailored to the situation at hand. Ethnic and cultural factors may play, also, a role in the perception and coping with the extreme stress.

Health and human service professionals need to direct their efforts to help older persons deal as constructively as possible with the psychological implications of their earlier stress experiences and social losses as well as aid their current adjustment. Older persons need to be respected within the structure and meaning of their social networks and associations since participation in social support networks is not only important for the availability of care in times of need, but also appears to promote a better state of mental health.

Although there are very clear differences between situations of extreme stress, these experiences place extraordinary demands on those who are forced to cope with their consequences and with the added challenges of aging. Not all survivors are debilitated by their earlier traumatic or extreme stressful experiences, however, some seek various forms of emotional and social support, and some seek individual and group therapy. It is important to underscore that we have limited understanding concerning sensitive and appropriate forms of therapy and support for survivors of extreme stress. It is important to acknowledge that many of the treatment approaches have limited empirical bases (Wilson et al., 1988).

The distress of the extreme stress survivor may often be shared in empathic ways by the therapist who has the responsibility to listen in non-judgmental ways about some of the most cruel, hideous and tortuous experiences that man has inflicted on his fellow man. The severity of the experiences may often create unique problems of counter-transference in the therapist (Danieli, 1980).

Evidence suggests that it is very unlikely that such massive psychic trauma may ever be assimilated or worked through. There is an ever present dynamic tension between wanting to forget and a need to remember with a particular vulnerability to loss and separation. Illness, hospitalization, institutionalization, social losses and other life stresses may reawaken earlier stress-related feelings of regimentation, helplessness and powerlessness. Among Holocaust survivors the recognition of the collective meaning of their experiences is also important.

It is important to recognize that working with survivors of extreme stress is challenging, difficult and emotionally taxing. And yet it must be kept in perspective that models for treatment of older survivors of extreme stress are only as useful as they aid their adjustment to current challenges and to consequences of their earlier stressful experiences. There is a potential danger to our clinical efforts if we uncritically accept treatment approaches based on unsubstantiated evidence. Research has begun to show that there are multiple patterns of coping with traumatic and extreme stress. Some have been deeply scarred and effected for the rest of their lives while other persons derived strength from their adversity and engaged in constructive and meaningful lives. Aiding the adjustment of survivors of traumatic and extreme stress will continue to challenge the genius of professional practice.

REFERENCES

Antonovsky, A. (1979). *Health, Stress and Coping.* San Francisco, CA: Jossey Bass.

Baider, L. & Sarell, M. (1984). Coping with cancer among Holocaust survivors in Israel: An exploratory study. *Journal of Stress,* 10, 121-128.

Ben-Sira, Z. (1985). Potency: A stress-buffering link in the coping-stress-disease relationship. *Social Science and Medicine,* 21 (4), 397-406.

Cohen, S. & Wills, T. A. (1985). Stress, social support, and the buffering hypothesis. *Psychological Bulletin,* 98 (2), 310-357.

Chodoff, P. (1963). Late effects of the Concentration Camp Syndrome. *Archives of General Psychiatry,* 8, 37-47.

Danieli, Y. (1980). Countertransference in the treatment and study of Nazi Holocaust survivors and their children. *Victimology: An International Journal,* 5, No. 2-4, pp. 355-367.

Dean, K. (1986). Social support and health: Pathways of influence. *Health Promotion,* 1 (2), 133-150.

DesPres, T. (1976). *The survivor: An anatomy of life in the death camps.* New York: Oxford University Press.

Eaton, W. W., Sigal, J. J., & Weinfeld, M. (1982). Impairment in Holocaust survivors after 33 years: Data from an unbiased community sample. *American Journal of Psychiatry*, 139 (6), pp. 773-777.

Elder, G. & Clip, E. (1988). Combat experience, comradeship, and psychological health. In J. P. Wilson, Z. Harel and B. Kahana (Eds.), *Human adaptation to extreme stress: From the Holocaust to Vietnam*. New York: Plenum.

Frankl, V. (1962). *Man's search for meaning: An introduction to Logotherapy*. Boston, MA: Beacon Press.

Galbraith, M. & Davison, D. (1985). Stress and elderly abuse. *Focus on Learning*, 11, 87-92.

Germain, C. (1978). General Systems Theory and Ego Psychology: An Ecological Perspective. *Social Service Review*, 52, pp. 535-550.

Gump, P. (1974). The Behavior Setting: A promising unit for environmental designers. In R. Moos & P. Insel (Eds.), *Issues in social ecology*. Palo Alto, CA: National Press Books, 267-275.

Harel, Z. (1988). Coping with extreme stress and aging. *Social Casework*, 575-583.

Harel, Z. & Deimling G. (1984). Social Resources and Mental Health: An Empirical Refinement. *Journal of Gerontology*, 39, 747-752.

Harel, Z., Kahana, B. & Kahana, E. (1984). Psychiatric, Behavioral Science and Survivor perspectives on the Holocaust. *Journal of Sociology and Social Welfare*, XI, 915-29.

Harel, Z., Kahana, B., & Kahana, E. (1988). Predictors of psychological well-being among Holocaust survivors and immigrants in Israel. *Journal of Traumatic Stress Studies*, 1, 413-429.

Harel, Z., Kahana, B. & Kahana, E. (1993). Social Resources and Mental Health of Aging Nazi Holocaust Survivors and Immigrants. In J. Wilson & B. Raphael (Eds.) *International Handbook of Traumatic Stress Syndromes*, New York: Plenum, pp. 241-252.

Harel, Z., Noelker, L. & Blake B. (1985). Planning Services for the Aged: Theoretical and Empirical Perspectives. *Gerontologist*, 25, 644-9.

Holahan C. J. & Moos, R. H. (1985). Life stress and health: Personality, coping and family support in stress resistance. *Journal of Personality & Social Psychology*, 49 (3), 739-747.

House, J. (1981). *Work Stress and Social Support*. Reading, MA: Addison-Wesley.

Jenkins, T., Parham, I. & Jenkins, L. (1985). Alzheimer's Disease: Caregivers' perception of burden. *Journal of Applied Gerontology*, 40-57.

Kahana, B., Harel, Z. & Kahana, E. (1989). Clinical and Gerontological Issues Facing Survivors of the Holocaust. In Marcus P. & Rosenberg, A. (Eds.), *Psychoanalytic reflections on the Holocaust*. New York: Praeger Publishers.

Kahana, E., Kahana, B., Harel, Z., & Rosner, T., (1988). Coping with Extreme Trauma. In Wilson, J., Harel, Z. & Kahana, B. (Eds.), *Human adaptation to extreme stress: From the Holocaust to Vietnam*. New York: Plenum Series on Stress.

Klein-Parker, F. (1988). Dominant attitudes of adult children of Holocaust survivors toward their parents. In J. P. Wilson, Z. Harel and B. Kahana (Eds.), *Human adaptation to extreme stress: From the Holocaust to Vietnam.* New York: Plenum.

Krause, N. (1987). Understanding the stress process: Linking social support with locus of control beliefs. *Journal of Gerontology*, 589-93.

Krystal, H. (1968). *Massive Psychic Trauma.* New York: International Universities Press.

Larson, R. (1978) Thirty years of research on the subjective well-being of older Americans. *Journal of Gerontology*, 40, pp. 109-129.

Lazarus, R., DeLongis, A., Folkman, S. & Gruen, R. (1985). Stress and adaptational outcomes: The problem of confounded measures. *American Psychologist*, 40 (7), 770-779.

Lazarus, R. S. & Folkman, S. (1984). *Stress, appraisal, and coping.* New York: Springer.

Noelker, L. & Harel, Z. (1983). The integration of environment and network theories in explaining the aged's functioning and well-being. *International Topics in Gerontology*, 17, 84-95. Basel, Switzerland: Karger.

Oswald, P. & Bittner, E. (1968). Life adjustment after severe persecution. *American Journal of Psychiatry*, 124, 87-94.

Palmore, J. (1979). Predictors of successful aging. *The Gerontologist*, 19, 427-431.

Rosenbloom, M. (1983). Implications of the Holocaust for social work. *Social Casework*, 64 (4), 205-213.

Sigal, J. J., Weinfeld, M. & Eaton, W. W. (1985). Stability of coping style 33 years after prolonged exposure to extreme stress. *Acta Psychiatrica Scandinavica*, 71 (6), 559-566.

Steinberg, A. (1989). Holocaust survivors and their children: A review of the clinical literature. In P. Marcus & A. Rosenberg (Eds.), *Psychoanalytic reflections on the Holocaust.* New York: Praeger Publishers.

Steinitz, L. Y. (1982). Psycho-social effects of the Holocaust on aging survivors and their families. *Journal of Gerontological Social Work*, 4 (3/4), 145-152.

Suls, J. & Fletcher, B. (1985). The relative efficacy of avoidant and nonavoidant coping strategies: A meta-analysis. *Health Psychology*, 4 (3), 249-288.

Wilson, J., Harel, Z., Kahana, B., Walker, A. & DeVaris D. (1988). The Day of Infamy 45 years later: Post-Traumatic response in Pearl Harbor survivors. In J. P. Wilson (Ed.), *Traumatic Stress: Theoretical and Clinical Implications.* New York: Bruner Mazel.

Wilson, J., Harel, Z. & Kahana, B. (Eds). (1988). *Human Adaptation to Extreme Stress: From the Holocaust to Vietnam.* New York: Plenum Series on Stress.

Heading Toward Normal:
Deinstitutionalization
for the Mentally Retarded Client

Craig Whitman

SUMMARY. "Heading Toward Normal: Deinstitutionalization for the Mentally Retarded Client" considers the differences between institutionalized and deinstitutionalized residential care for people who are mentally challenged. Normalization is presented as a method to include people who are disabled in culturally normative activities.

A project associated with deinstitutionalization for two subjects is described and the results of psychological tests are given. The conclusion of the study suggests that socialization opportunities within the community play a significant role in the personal development of individuals with developmental disabilities.

INTRODUCTION

How to best care for mentally retarded persons has been a long-standing dilemma. Some reasons for their isolation have included fear by the general public of people who are different and the difficulty with which to provide for the needs of handicapped individuals. Large institutions accommodating several hundred mentally retarded residents, and more recently smaller group homes, have

---

Craig Whitman is Clinical Director for Catholic Community Services, Bisbee, AZ, and Associate Faculty Member, Cochise College, Douglas, AZ.

[Haworth co-indexing entry note]: "Heading Toward Normal: Deinstitutionalization for the Mentally Retarded Client." Whitman, Craig. Co-published simultaneously in *Marriage & Family Review* (The Haworth Press, Inc.) Vol. 21, No. 1/2, 1995, pp. 51-64; and: *Exemplary Social Intervention Programs for Members and Their Families* (ed: David Guttmann, and Marvin B. Sussman) The Haworth Press, Inc., 1995, pp. 51-64. Multiple copies of this article/chapter may be purchased from The Haworth Document Delivery Center [1-800-3-HAWORTH; 9:00 a.m. - 5:00 p.m. (EST)].

51

served as the placements of choice during the twentieth century. Institutionalized settings were viewed as having several advantages for the care of mentally retarded and otherwise handicapped individuals by alleviating the burden of responsibility from the residents' parents and creating a community of people who were presumably similar in significant ways. Society was equally considered in that fears pertaining to people who were different were addressed by isolating these individuals and removing them from public view and traditional places of residence.

One presumed advantage of institutional living for mentally challenged persons was a sense of commonality with respect to the social adaptability and levels of functioning of the residents. Simply put, the institution was created to reflect the skills of the residents and therefore make it easy for them to feel comfortable within the walls of the institution. Medical care was also provided on site and therefore those residents with severe medical needs could be attended to readily. Activities and academic training for people with handicaps could also be designed to mirror the true levels of skill and development of the residents. Vocational opportunities and the teaching of vocational skills could also be provided on site.

INSTITUTIONALIZATION VERSUS DEINSTITUTIONALIZATION

The picture that the author has described about institutions is a most optimistic one and it is only in the late twentieth century that institutions for the mentally retarded evolved to the humanistic stage that has been presented. In the more distant past, warehousing was reflective of the most primitive instincts of society and it was less an issue of providing for the mentally retarded residents and more of an attempt to protect society from what may have appeared to be contagious and dangerous. The risks involved in institutionalization, despite the goal of creating a common culture for people with common problems, include depersonalization.

The Arizona Department of Economic Security (DES), Division of Developmental Disabilities (DDD), expresses in its "Statement of Rights" the following guidelines:

> Every developmentally disabled individual who is provided residential care by the state shall have the right to live in the least restrictive alternative, as determined after an initial placement evaluation has been conducted for such individual.

> Developmentally disabled individuals who are in residential programs operated or supported by the Department, shall have the right to humane and clean physical environment, the right to communication and visits, and the right to personal property (1983, 1).

The idea that people who are mentally retarded, or more globally the developmentally disabled, have rights is a monumental development. The pursuit of the "least restrictive environment," suggesting "the utilization of means which are as culturally normative as possible in order to establish and/or maintain personal behaviors and characteristics which are as culturally normative as possible" (Arizona Department of Economic Security, 1983, 1), is a breakthrough of enormous consequence.

Previously, mentally challenged and disabled people were removed from the mainstream of society and, for the sake of their protection or others', were isolated in facilities for their care. In *Understanding Mental Retardation* (1986) Zigler and Hodapp chronicle the ebb and flow of the institutionalization and deinstitutionalization movements. In essence, some of the issues most pertinent to these movements include:

A. Can mentally retarded people learn?
B. Are mentally retarded people dangerous to others?
C. Should mentally retarded people be isolated from or integrated into society?

The advent of the National Association for Retarded Children (NARC) in 1951, and the Civil Rights Movement during the 1960s created a climate of reform that contributed to the development of deinstitutionalization (DiGregorio, 1986). In 1971, the Partlow facility in Alabama was in jeopardy of dramatic reductions in funding and thus a new focus upon community treatment began. The proposition that mentally retarded people had the ability to succeed and would be better served outside the confines of the institution was a controversial one.

Normalization pushed deinstitutionalization to its limits. Bengt Nirje (DeWeaver, 1983, 435) described normalization as a method of providing common and typical experiences to handicapped people that are available to members of the society at large. The author has often thought that it is impossible to teach people normal behavior without exposing them to normal situations. The mentally challenged person with limited cognitive ability may never achieve a level of functioning equal to those of normal ability; nevertheless, exposure to typical, common, everyday occurrences creates the possibility and the opportunity for abnormal people to behave normally. This possibility speaks against the advantages of isolation that exist in institutionalized settings, including group homes. It is frequently acknowledged that prisoners serving time in prisons receive an education in the form of socialization with other prisoners that leads them to become better criminals. The isolation of mentally challenged persons from the larger society has impact upon their ability to expand developmentally, model normal behavior, and reap the satisfaction of learning new skills that are useful to them in a larger world.

A PERSONAL EXPERIENCE

In 1972 the Willowbrook institution in New York City, one that the author visited at that time, was sued for a variety of reasons. Eighty percent of the school-aged children received no education whatsoever, and ninety-six percent of the adult residents received no educational programming. In addition to the above, one hundred percent of all residents contracted hepatitis within six months of entering the institution, and scabies, pneumonia and roaches were present in epidemic proportions (Zigler and Hodapp, 1986).

Following an exposé by Geraldo Rivera in 1972 which showed residents sitting unattended in large, bare, sterile rooms, banging their heads upon the walls, the author visited Willowbrook in Staten Island to see firsthand what the institution was like. The author attempted to be unobtrusive to gain the most accurate picture of life there, and found himself joining a group of approximately ten residents being led across the grassy grounds to lunch. No one attempted to question the author as to why he was there. The author was immediately struck by the high level of stress reflected in the expression of the one staff person leading the group toward the lunch building. As the author sat with the group, there was no apparent interaction or verbal communication among the residents. The staff person seemed somewhat overwhelmed with his role of being responsible for his many charges, and treated the residents as a group to be herded, rather than with any individuation. The feeling that the author had about the entire experience was that it was a routine intended to be completed as quickly and systematically as possible without any genuine investment toward enjoyment or training.

Biklen (1979) points out that the turnover among employees at institutions is extremely high and that residents are likely to be cared for by hundreds of different staff over a two or three year period rather than a few primary caregivers. Given the nature of the Willowbrook institutionalized setting at that time and the role expectations for staff and resident alike, it would appear that each conformed to the institutionalized model suggested by Wolfensberger:

> It is a well-established fact that a person's behavior tends to be profoundly affected by the role expectations that are placed upon him . . . people will play the roles that they have been assigned. This permits those who define social roles to make self-fulfilling prophesies by predicting that someone cast into certain roles will emit behavior consistent with that role. Unfortunately, role-appropriate behavior will then often be interpreted to be a person's "natural" rather than elicited mode of action (Wolfensberger, 1976, 36).

The residents that the author observed at Willowbrook did not reflect any individuation due to the setting's discouragement of such individuation.

A DEINSTITUTIONALIZED RESIDENTIAL MODEL

In 1986 the author left his position as case manager for the Division of Developmental Disabilities, a position that the author had held for over four years. A mentally retarded man whose pseudonym will be Thomas was placed in the author's home and so began the author's new role as an adult developmental home provider; this is similar to being a foster parent for adults who have developmental disabilities. Thomas was 53 years old, African-American, and had been diagnosed as being in the profound/low range of mental retardation. Thomas had grown up living in a large institution for the mentally retarded and had subsequently been placed in a group home in recent years.

In 1987 the author made arrangements with the Division of Developmental Disabilities to place Lenny, also a pseudonym, in a vacant house next door to the author's home. This was a highly unusual arrangement since it is so atypical for a residential provider to live next door to his/her client. Lenny was 40 years old, white, and had been diagnosed as mildly mentally retarded. The author expected that with assistance Lenny could learn to live semi-independently in his own home due to his high level of functioning. Despite Lenny's high potential, he also presented a series of emotional problems and dysfunctional behaviors including sexual exposure, cross-dressing, lying, stealing and hostile emotional outbursts. The author hoped that Lenny could be integrated into the community as a result of his abilities and the author's supervision.

In 1988 the author moved Thomas next door into Lenny's home. Both men had lived together previously in their former group home and had gotten along quite well. The difference in their levels of functioning did not appear to interfere with the friendship that had developed between them, and each man expressed positive sentiments toward becoming housemates again. The author viewed the opportunity for Thomas to live in his own house following a lifetime of institutionalization as a tremendous step in the direction of personal development and normalization. Despite Thomas' mostly nonverbal way of communicating, he made it clear to the author and others that he reveled in the opportunity to live in his own home independent of staff. On one occasion prior to Thomas' move next door with Lenny, he pointed out to the author that he too wanted his own house. Thomas was aware that the author had his house, Lenny had his house, and Thomas pointed in the direction of another house that he would have liked as his own. Under ordinary circumstances

Thomas could never share a home with his friend, Lenny, without the continuous monitoring by staff that is so much a part of institutional life. Due to the unique arrangement of Lenny's and the author's houses and the extended family relationship among all concerned, Thomas was given the opportunity to live semi-independently.

For Lenny's part, he viewed Thomas as an excellent companion who would not intrude upon his privacy. Lenny was a very expansive person who appreciated a considerable amount of space for his projects such as building with wood, using power tools, maintaining his dog and three cats, watching television and listening to music. Since Thomas tended to prefer to be in his own room as a sort of sanctuary, Lenny had free reign of the house and an unobtrusive companion nearby for company. Lenny felt the satisfaction of inviting Thomas to share his home and simultaneously he raised his sense of self-esteem by looking after someone who was less capable than himself.

As the men began to live together, they became more and more expressive of a culture that reflected their unique personalities. Thomas, for example, enjoyed being taken to the library while Lenny remained at home to work on a project with his tools. Lenny would request to be taken to the lumber yard while Thomas arranged his magazine collection and sang songs and hymns in his room. Since Thomas was considerably more dependent and lower functioning than Lenny, the author continued to supervise his meals and many other activities while giving him the satisfaction of living in his own home. Lenny prepared his own meals. Lenny was also free to go out to eat by himself on weekends while Thomas and the author would engage in community activities together. In effect, the "one to two" staff to client supervision ratio and the flexibility with which client needs were met encouraged a highly personalized program. This staff to client ratio even improved as the author's fiancée, Holly, and her nine-year-old daughter, Kara, became more and more-involved. Today we are a family, and we serve as Lenny's and Thomas' extended family as well.

SOME EXAMPLES OF PROGRESS

To document progress in areas in which training is being provided to developmentally disabled clients, the Individual Program

Plan (IPP) is implemented. The IPP intends to specify training that is needed by mentally challenged people who are clients of the social services system. The very nature of the training areas, or "objectives," of the IPP reinforces the author's belief that people are circumscribed by their socialization opportunities. A person who is mentally retarded will not be taught how to use public transportation if he/she has no access to such transportation due to the confines of the institution or group home. It is only in normalized circumstances that individuals will be expected to learn skills associated with normalcy.

Lenny entered his current semi-independent living arrangement with objectives focused upon learning to cook parts of a meal and making small purchases within the community. Both of these objectives were developed at Lenny's former group home and required staff supervision. Today Lenny prepares all of his meals independently. He is responsible for developing a weekly grocery shopping list that is written with the assistance of the author. Lenny surveys the supermarket shelves and selects the items himself. He has become an individual person and no longer behaves as part of an institutional group home of five or six residents.

With regard to making small purchases within the community, this former objective has been modified in several ways. First, staff is no longer present when these purchases are made. Second, Lenny gets on and off public transportation whenever necessary to make purchases; this differs from traveling with other group home clients in a van belonging to the group home. Last, Lenny now has access to go to restaurants on weekends and goes out to eat independently.

Another observable change in Lenny that has developed due to the personal investment of the residential provider and his wife, Holly, has been Lenny's improved attitude and a diminishment of his dysfunctional behavior. As in the case of anyone experiencing "recovery issues" (Alcoholics Anonymous, Co-dependents Anonymous, etc.), honesty with oneself and toward others is mandatory if any genuine change is to transpire. Lenny has had many "slips" since his arrival in 1987 with regard to sexual exposure, stealing, lying and emotional outbursts. Nevertheless, true progress has been made regarding all of these behaviors and Lenny has reached an inner equilibrium that reflects a happier, more trustworthy person. The author believes that it has been the proximity of our lives in the forms of being neighbors and extended family members that has enabled Holly and the author to hold Lenny accountable for his behavior and give him the emotional support that he has needed for change.

Thomas moved into the author's home in 1986 and moved next door with Lenny in 1988. When Thomas arrived, he was primarily nonverbal and communicated his needs through gestures; for example, he would point at foods in the refrigerator when he was hungry and point to his groinal area when he needed to urinate. Over time Thomas began to articulate what he wanted. This was primarily due to the author's requirement that Thomas attempt to express himself verbally. It was quite astounding how many words Thomas could say if given the opportunity to do so. Since Thomas' arrival, the author and many people within the community have remarked how much more communicative and understandable he has become.

Thomas has also taken to robustly singing songs and hymns in his room. Holly and the author believe that Thomas is expressing an inner joy that has come from feeling cared about by a consistent extended family that he has never had previously during his many years of institutionalization. Apparently, Thomas was socialized to learn many songs and hymns during his lifetime. It is the deep expression of "being home" and his newfound sense of the freedom to be himself that the author finds so truly moving. This type of freedom is often sorely missing in institutional settings that must conform its standards to the needs of the group at any given time.

An unusual example of Thomas' progress associated with his deinstitutionalized residential placement occurred in November, 1993. A postcard reminding the patient of his semi-annual dental cleaning was sent by the dentist accidentally to Thomas' vocational program instead of to Thomas' home. The vocational staff at the sheltered workshop explained to Thomas what the postcard was for and gave Thomas the postcard. He was instructed to bring the postcard home to Holly and the author so that they could arrange his appointment. What happened next was truly remarkable.

On his way home from work that day, Thomas informed the bus driver that he needed to go to the dentist, showing him the postcard. He had seen Lenny get on and off the city bus many times to attend dental appointments. Thomas got off the city bus and walked a short distance to the dentist's office. Thomas informed the dentist's staff that he needed to make an appointment for his cleaning. The dentist's staff provided Thomas with an appointment to have his teeth cleaned. Once this task was completed, Thomas walked over a mile to his home and informed Holly and the author of where he had been and what had been done for him, giving them the small business card confirming the appointment. Holly and the author called the dentist's office to confirm what it seemed Thomas had communicated. Although deeply concerned due to Thomas' disappearance after work, Holly and the author praised Thomas for his initiative and competence and marvelled at just how far he had come since moving into semi-independent living.

To summarize the primary qualities that distinguish this residential program and its attempt to promote successful individuation for the clients involved, here are the most significant aspects: (a) the two adults with mental retardation live in their own house and their residential provider, the author, lives next door in his house; this is a highly unusual arrangement and the author has been told by several staff from the Division of Developmental Disabilities that it is unique in the state of Arizona; (b) the residential provider and his family have created a family-like relationship with the clients without living in the same house; this varies from adult foster care in which the clients are part of a family while living in the family's home; (c) the residential provider and his family provide ongoing supervision throughout the week, unlike institutionalized settings that have staff rotating on shifts; (d) unlike other residential models, there has been no staff turnover since the program's inception over seven and one-half years ago; (e) the residential provider has a Ph.D. degree in social work and provides a therapeutic as well as a functional relationship for the clients; this means that the author and his wife intervene and address Lenny's previously described dysfunctional behaviors through an ongoing counseling relationship that occurs within the deinstitutionalized context of daily living.

PSYCHOLOGICAL TESTS

The author's purpose in sharing the results of psychological assessments is to provide a comparative analysis that will offer insight into the trends pertaining to Thomas and Lenny's personal growth. Although it may be difficult to assume that there is an exact correlation between changes in Thomas and Lenny's levels of functioning and their changes in residential placement, the author believes that the results of their prior and more recent psychological tests do give a good indication of how the process of deinstitutionalization has impacted upon their performance.

In September of 1971, Thomas was assessed an I.Q. score of 13 in relation to the administration of the Peabody Picture Vocabulary Test (P.P.V.T.). This score placed Thomas in the profound/low severe range of mental retardation. An "Updated Psychological Summary" (undated) referred to the 1971 P.P.V.T. and commented that, "An earlier assessment (Binet completed in 1964), also was consistent with the above findings."

In September of 1990, the results of the Vineland Social Maturity Scale indicated that Thomas' diagnosis is "moderate mental retardation or high end of severe retardation." A second administration of the Vineland Social Maturity Scale, using the author as the informant about Thomas' abilities revealed similar results in October of 1990. Thus, since 1971 Thomas' documented level of mental retardation has changed from profound/low severe, usually described as being totally dependent upon others for survival, to moderate/high severe, usually associated with some degree of independent living as well as a protected environment. During this period of time, Thomas was moved from institutional living in a large institution to group home living in 1982 and more recently to more personalized residential services in 1986.

In Lenny's case, the results are equally startling. In June of 1980 the Vineland Social Maturity Scale indicated that Lenny's age equivalent was 6 years and 9 months. In October of 1990 the Vineland evaluation, using the author as the source of information, determined that Lenny's age equivalent was exactly 10 years. The Diagnostic Statement and Summary at the end of the 1980 examination suggested that Lenny "appears to be functioning in the mild range of mental retardation. . . ." Another Vineland evaluation in September of 1990 states that Lenny "functions at a high level of Mild Mental Retardation." Thus, keeping in mind that Lenny moved from a large institution to group home living in 1984, followed by his move into his own house in 1987, it appears that these changes in residential setting have contributed positively toward Lenny's level of functioning and intelligence.

CONCLUSION

The nature of residential care for people who are mentally challenged has changed considerably during the twentieth century. These changes have been the result of changing attitudes reflective of a more humane approach to the residential needs of this unique population.

When considering the process of deinstitutionalization for the mentally retarded client, the concept of normalization immediately comes to mind. "The normalization principle means making available to all mentally retarded people patterns of life and conditions of everyday living which are as close as possible to the regular circumstances and ways of life of society" (Nirje qtd. in DeWeaver, 1983, 435).

The concept of normalization is a quantum leap for the treatment of the mentally retarded person. We are no longer solely reflecting upon whether the disabled person is receiving adequate care to meet his/her basic needs; rather the discussion now revolves around a socialization process aimed at creating opportunities for the handicapped to be integrated into society.

Following the advent of institutional settings intended to safeguard the welfare of people who were developmentally disabled, a reevaluation occurred consistent with an enlightened attempt to promote client rights. The personal growth and enlargement of skills associated with deinstitutionalization became paramount factors in determining what is truly in the best interests of the individual. Group homes and semi-independent apartment programs evolved in answer to the changing needs of this client-population; however, the author believes that there is more yet to be done.

The project described within this study developed in stages beginning in 1986. The momentum of the project always aimed toward greater independence for the two participants involved. Thomas' movement from a group home to an adult developmental home in which he lived with the author was a monumental step. Thomas' further movement into his own home with Lenny far exceeded previous expectations held by staff who knew him as an institutional or a group home resident. The results of Thomas' psychological tests reflect personal growth and greater cognitive ability that parallel his residential moves.

Despite Lenny's emotional problems, he had the potential to learn many skills that would support him in semi-independent living. Lenny has truly grown in competence since moving into his own home and his psychological test results are consistent with that growth. Lenny's mobility within the community and his access to public transportation, restaurants and community residents was severely limited while he lived in a large institution and subsequently a group home. Since moving into his own home in 1987 Lenny has become a more communicative person who expresses his wants and needs and has the local community as a context through which he may meet those needs.

The socialization process provided through institutionalization, whether it is a large institution or a smaller group home, is immediately circumscribed within the parameters of the setting. The institutionalized mentally retarded resident can never be expected to learn behavior that may only be found outside of the facility; therefore the process of normalization will extend only insofar as the institution resembles the outside world. It is the author's belief that living in one's own home is a critical dynamic that contributes to greater competence and maturity. Having a residential provider living next door allows the client to experience a genuine sense of independence without losing a support system that is vital.

Socialization is the process by which we become full participants in society (Conklin, 1987). Normalization is the socialization process applied to people with developmental disabilities. Lenny and Thomas have shown that people who are mentally challenged can exceed expectations if they are given exposure to normal circumstances such as living in one's own home and becoming part of a community.

REFERENCES

Arizona Department of Economic Security (1983). *Mission statement.*
Biklen, D. (1979). The case for deinstitutionalization. *Social Policy, 10,* 48-54.
Conklin, J. (1987). *Sociology: An introduction.* New York: Macmillan Publishing Company.

DeWeaver, K. (1983). Deinstitutionalization of the developmentally disabled. *Social Work, 28* (6), 435-39.

DiGregorio, J. (1983). *A psychological investigation of deinstitutionalization.* Cincinnati: The Union Graduate School.

Rivera, G. (1972). Television news.

Wolfensberger, W. (1972). *The principle of normalization in human services.* Toronto: National Institute on Mental Retardation.

Zigler, E. and Hodapp, R. (1986). *Understanding mental retardation.* Cambridge: Cambridge University Press.

Working with Poor Families– Lessons Learned from Practice

Marsha R. Mueller
Michael Q. Patton

SUMMARY. This article describes lessons learned from practice; lessons learned about how generally accepted guiding principles are translated into effective work with poor families. This article is based on the diverse experiences and evaluations of seven effective parenting/family stability programs which were part of The McKnight Foundation's Families in Poverty initiative. A major focus of this article is on program dynamics and interconnections; characteristics of effectiveness and lessons learned from practice which cut across all seven programs. Programming themes emphasized the importance of mission, responsiveness, flexibility, comprehensive delivery strategies, and knowledge management.

INTRODUCTION

The concept of working comprehensively with whole families has received increased attention by practitioners, poverty experts,

---

Marsha R. Mueller is a social scientist and independent evaluation consultant. She earned her Master's degree from the Department of Social Science, University of Chicago. Michael Q. Patton is a social scientist, evaluator, and futurist.

This article is based on the synthesis evaluation of The McKnight Foundation's Families in Poverty initiative; a five-year evaluation effort funded by The McKnight Foundation.

[Haworth co-indexing entry note]: "Working with Poor Families–Lessons Learned from Practice." Mueller, Marsha R., and Michael Q. Patton. Co-published simultaneously in *Marriage & Family Review* (The Haworth Press, Inc.) Vol. 21, No. 1/2, 1995, pp. 65-90; and: *Exemplary Social Intervention Programs for Members and Their Families* (ed: David Guttmann, and Marvin B. Sussman) The Haworth Press, Inc., 1995, pp. 65-90. Multiple copies of this article/chapter may be purchased from The Haworth Document Delivery Center [1-800-3-HAWORTH; 9:00 a.m. - 5:00 p.m. (EST)].

65

and policy makers. Considerable work has been devoted over the past decade to family approaches by public and private initiatives (see Kagan, Powell, Weissbourd, & Zigler, 1987; Schorr, 1988; Weiss & Jacobs, 1988). The results of this work show ". . . a convergence as to *guiding principles:* programs should be family focused, holistic, community-based, consumer-oriented, culturally sensitive, comprehensive, and integrated or coordinated to create a system of care" (Kahn & Kamerman, 1992). As interest in family issues and family focused programs increases, so does the list of practical questions about what can be expected from family programs. However, as Weiss and Halpern (1990) note, family support programs, given their predominately local sponsorship, rarely have the resources to systematically evaluate their effectiveness. As a result, the empirical base of information is limited–practice outpaces research.

The purpose of this article is to describe lessons learned from practice; lessons learned about *how* rhetoric becomes reality–*how* generally accepted guiding principles are translated into effective work with poor families. This article is based on the diverse experiences and evaluations of seven effective parenting/family stability programs which were part of The McKnight Foundation's Families in Poverty (FIP) initiative.

The McKnight Foundation's Families in Poverty (FIP) Initiative

The FIP initiative represents a comprehensive approach by The McKnight Foundation to respond to severe economic and social trends developing in the 1980s, which limited the ability of both governments and nonprofit human service systems to address the needs of poor families (McKnight, 1991). One focus of this initiative was to strengthen family stability and improve parenting skills. In 1988, McKnight made grants to seven effective parenting/family stability programs as part of the Foundation's $13 million initiative. The other FIP clusters included employment, child care, and comprehensive programs. In total, FIP included 34 projects.

The Foundation's purpose was not solely to help participating families, as important as that was, but to have a broader impact by learning about strategies that work, and those that do not. The significance of The McKnight Foundation's approach and the impact of its involvement in the FIP initiative on participants and program outcomes is discussed elsewhere (see Patton, 1993). What is important to note here is that the Foundation set the tone for the initiative ". . . by the way it funded, administered, and supported program grants." The bottom line message was: *Do whatever makes sense to help families get out of poverty* (Patton, 1993).

The initiative was not conceived as a tightly controlled research and demonstration project. The Foundation encouraged staffs to adapt their strategies to changed circumstances and to redesign approaches when they were found to be ineffective. Original targets for recruiting participants or making progress toward proposed benchmarks became less important than uncovering participant issues, setting individualized and realistic goals, and learning from practice (McKnight, 1991).

McKnight managed accountability by emphasizing learning and supporting an interactive evaluation system which included project level evaluations, cluster evaluations, and a comprehensive synthesis (see Illustration 1). Each project was responsible for evaluating their work and submitting annual reports to the Foundation. The Foundation supported this expectation through funding for evaluation and providing evaluation training. In addition, annual FIP conferences were convened by McKnight to discuss lessons learned from program and evaluation efforts.

Project evaluations formed the core focus of the initiative's evaluation team. The initiative evaluation team was responsible for synthesizing over-arching themes, patterns and lessons learned that cut across separate FIP programs and clusters. The team examined patterns of participant outcomes, program implementation themes, the ways program staffs worked with participants, larger impacts on agencies that hosted programs, governmental approaches and policy changes.

The evaluation was not driven by public accountability concerns about taking credit or assigning blame. Nor was a research methodology used to impress academic audiences. The mandate was to collect, credible data that would provide feedback for program improvement and document lessons learned.

ILLUSTRATION 1

FIP EVALUATION SYSTEM

---

32 Individual Grant Progress Reports and Evaluations

Each grant was responsible for its own program evaluation.

Four Cluster Evaluations

● 11 Comprehensive programs ● 6 Employment programs ● 8 Child care programs
● 7 Effective parenting/family stability programs

Each cluster evaluation includes:
  (a) a technical summary of each grant in the cluster, and
  (b) an overview synthesis of patterns and themes for the cluster.

OVERALL FIP SYNTHESIS EVALUATION

Includes patterns and themes across all four clusters:

● *Interconnections from a systems perspective*
● *Types of outcomes attained and specific outcome themes*
● *Programming and implementation themes*
● *System change themes*
● *Lessons about evaluation*

Intended Users and Potential Audiences at EACH Level

The McKnight Foundation; FIP grantees; and people locally and nationally making decisions about, delivering, and evaluating family poverty programs.

FIP Effective Parenting/Family Stability Programs

The seven effective parenting/family stability programs represent seven different approaches to family support. As a group, these programs worked with 1,145 families from 1988-1991. In all cases, participation in a project was voluntary and participants were acquired in different ways. Clientele were defined, for example, low income parents with young children in a geographically defined neighborhood, or students and their families from a specific school, and channels for accepting referrals identified. The length of time participants remained with a program as well as the intensity of their involvement varied. Overall, a majority of the families, over 75%, had substantial contact: families developed working relationships with program staff; took advantage of program services; and participated to the extent that progress could be assessed.

Participant Characteristics and Issues

The typical participant family was headed by an unemployed female who had not achieved a high school diploma, had an income under $10,000, and was an ethnic minority. Four programs reported that families of color accounted for a majority of participants. Three projects served multiple ethnic groups (African American, Caucasian, Native American, Asian, and Hispanic). One program served a specific population group: the Black Family Parent Education project focused on African Americans served by Black churches.

Challenges participating families faced included such life support issues as insufficient income, lack of adequate transportation, problems securing safe housing or food, and access to medical services. Other issues were parent problems including abuse or conflict between adults or physical or mental health problems; parenting issues around inconsistencies in applying rules and discipline, physical abuse or neglect and difficulty getting along with children. Child issues included school performance, aggressiveness/impulsive behavior, school attendance, sibling/peer relations, physical and mental health problems. Many families also faced legal problems and experienced social isolation. Most programs reported that the number of severely disadvantaged families served increased from 1988-1991.

Staffs found that the families they worked with were more unique than similar and the issues families faced were more complex than anticipated. Participant diversity and issue complexity were key themes from evaluation reports, site visits, and staff comments on implementation experiences. This is significant since most project staff had been working with people in poverty a long time. Most staffs reported that the emphasis on families and family strengths required more information than traditional work with individuals.

Systematic means of assessing family issues were used when families became involved. Some staffs used information from assessments conducted by other human service professionals to supplement their own data collection efforts. For example, one project used information collected by Public Health nurses in conjunction with enrollment data collected by staff.

Assessments of family situations were not a one-time event. In most programs it was an ongoing process. Trust had to be developed to go beyond surface appearances to fundamental issues and family strengths. It takes time to understand enough about a family's dynamics to put together a meaningful plan or working relationship. Effective staff learned to balance inquiry about problems with questions about participants' own perceptions about solutions. Needs assessment was balanced by assets analysis; and identification of weaknesses was matched by attention to strengths.

Project Descriptions and Major Outcomes

The following summaries note the project's primary purpose, key operating assumptions, delivery strategies, number of participants reached during the first three years, evaluation approaches and major outcomes.

St. Joseph's Home for Children: Effective Parenting Family Stability Program. This program provides intensive, short-term intervention with multiproblem families. Intervention specialists work over a twelve week period, with four to six families whose children have been placed at the Hennepin County emergency shelter, to prevent future shelter placements. The purpose of the project is to help stabilize the family environment, sort out issues, engage family members in problem-solving and help families to understand their own unique strengths. The primary assumption is that intensive, short-term intervention is an effective means of strengthening families and preventing repeat placements of children in St. Joseph's emergency shelter.

Staff worked with an external evaluator to design and implement a process and outcome evaluation. The outcome evaluation uses a constructed control group design and assesses effectiveness in reducing shelter recidivism rates and compares program costs to shelter stays. The process evaluation makes use of detailed records kept by each intervention specialist. The records include family intake information and preliminary measures of seventeen categories of family issues, weekly progress assessments, services provided and hours of direct contact with families, the twelve-week termination assessment, and three-month follow-up interview.

During the first three years the program served 144 families. Shelter readmission rates were found to be lower for program participants than for the shelter control group, 15% compared to 22%, three months following program participation. In addition, 76.9% of participating families demonstrated progress and improvement in issues identified at intake. Such progress included improvement in the area of motivation for problem-solving; a decrease in the use of physical punishment; improved knowledge of child care and development; strengthened family support systems; improved supervision of children; improvement in their financial situation; better ability to provide for the physical needs of children; and improved parenting skills, use of verbal discipline, and quality of parent-child relationships.

St. Paul Public Schools, Ramsey County Public Health Nursing Service, Payne-Phalen District 5 Council: Payne-Phalen Family Support Project. The Payne-Phalen Family Support Project is a neighborhood-based program providing information and support to families with children from birth to kindergarten. The project offers parenting education and support through home visits and at a neighborhood drop-in center. The purpose is to provide services to families that empower and strengthen adults in their roles as parents, nurturers and providers. Strategies are based on the following assumptions: all families need information and support for the parenting role; all families have strengths and parents need help that identifies and builds on these strengths; a variety of family forms can promote the healthy development of children and adults; and cultural differences and diversity are valid and valuable.

The program's director designed and implemented the evaluation. Preliminary consultation on the design was provided by Moncrieff Cochran, Director of the Family Empowerment Project, Cornell University. The evaluation makes use of comprehensive baseline measures for home visited families, participation data for both home visited and drop-in families, and one year follow-up interviews. In addition, a community survey was conducted during the third year of program operation to evaluate community satisfaction with the program.

The program worked with 267 referral families that received home visits and an additional 250 neighborhood "drop-in" families that participated in center activities. This program is successful in involving low income families in an ethnically diverse neighborhood; many adults in those families subsequently enroll in and complete a range of educational programs, and some adults gain employment. The program has successfully engaged severely disadvantaged families in both home visit and center activities. Evaluation findings report that families who are experiencing multiple, complex issues use the Family Resource Center at a higher rate than other home visited families. The program is also successful in reducing isolation. At the time of referral, over 50% of families report feeling alone or socially isolated; on follow-up interviews most report they have someone to talk to about parenting and child-rearing concerns. This project became the model for other family resource centers that now exist in St. Paul.

Merriam Park Community Center, Hallie Q. Brown/Martin Luther King Center, Longfellow Humanities Magnet School City of St. Paul: Early Intervention Poverty Prevention Program. This program helps grade school children develop healthy problem-solving skills through participation in small group sessions. Four to ten students meet weekly for an hour or less, throughout the school year, under the leadership of two skilled social worker teams. In addition, children may participate in a summer program. Social skill development is stressed using behavior modification methods, including discussion of personal concerns and clarification of values about attitudinal and behavioral alternatives. Also provided was support for families. This includes parent support groups, individual and family counseling, home visits as requested, and family oriented recreational activities. This project is based on the assumption that the best way to prevent teen pregnancies, chemical dependency, and delinquency is by assisting elementary age youngsters to clarify and set appropriate values by which their adult lives will be guided.

An external evaluator designed and conducted a process evaluation. The evaluation included teacher and parent ratings of child behavior at the beginning and end of the school year, group interviews with teachers, case notes, group leader summaries, and child self-assessments. In addition, both project and control group children were tracked by the school district to evaluate differences in pregnancy rates, drug use, school performance, retention, and criminal behavior.

One hundred eighty children were served during the first three years of the program. Children demonstrated these behavioral improvements: ability to attend to task, resolve conflicts, and enhanced social skills. Children who participated for three consecutive years demonstrated improved leadership abilities in school. Staff learned that effective school/community partnerships are built over time and require active participation and flexibility.

Survival Skills Institute, Inc.: The Black Family Parenting Education Project. The Black Family Parenting Education Project is designed to empower Black churches to provide parenting education to at-risk African-American parents who are either church members or reside in the community where the church is located. The program provides training to church-based instructors who in turn implement a 20-week parent class. Both instructor training and the parent education classes are supported by culturally relevant curriculums developed by Survival Skills Institute. The basic assumption of this program is that life outcomes for Black families are improved by strengthening the role church communities play in the lives of Black families.

The program contracted with an external evaluator. During the first year a survey and group interviews with church leaders were conducted as well as a review of participant demographics. During the second year, in addition to church leader interviews, participants' knowledge of parenting concepts were evaluated based on pre- and post-program assessments. During year three group interviews were held with participants and church leaders and a survey of past participants was conducted. In addition to discussing major outcomes, the final report includes a literature review on African-American parenting and family research.

Four churches were actively involved through the first three years and served 160 families. Participants demonstrated knowledge gains: the average gain per curriculum unit was 14.8 points on a 100-point grading scale. The typical participant did not possess the required minimal knowledge at the beginning of the unit but was able to demonstrate knowledge competency on tests following each unit. Parents also reported improved parenting practices as a result of their participation in the program.

Episcopal Community Services: Family To Family Ties. Family To Family Ties matches a family in need with church volunteer families. Volunteer families are trained to provide information and ongoing support to assist participant families in taking charge of their lives. The target population for this program are low income families, many of whom are single parents needing ongoing support and guidance as well as food, clothing, and shelter. The approach is designed as a partnership and is based on the assumption that volunteer and participant families can learn from each other. This program applied for a one-year grant and later received a second-year grant. By the end of year two, 28 participant families were matched with 36 volunteer families from 15 churches.

The program budget did not allow for the development of a systematic evaluation plan. However, the program was informally evaluated by staff. Their efforts included an evaluation of volunteer training sessions, interviews with families and volunteers every six months, and reviews of program records. Feedback from participants and volunteers indicated that the program was successful in helping families acquire new parenting and financial management skills. In addition, volunteers reported new understanding about poverty issues.

Columbia Heights Early Childhood Family Education: At-Home, On-Site Parent Education Program. This program provides educational services to families with young children ages birth through pre-kindergarten. Participants are referred to the program from several sources: public health nurses; day care licensing; child protection; and the Way to Grow House. Home educators visit participants and use a variety of teaching methods to enhance parenting skills. A typical hour and a half visit is divided between direct activity time with a child using materials brought by the home educator and discussion with the parent.

A different evaluator was retained each year. The final report is based on a case file review, follow-up interviews with former participants, a summary of parent demographic characteristics, and a review of the first two evaluation reports.

During the project's three years, home educators worked with 65 families to enhance parenting skills: parenting skills improved for a majority of families; parents who received 20 or more visits became more aware of community services; and one-third of the program parents enrolled in school-based Early Childhood Family Education classes.

Anoka County Community Action Program, Inc.: Project Independence. Project Independence was a case management program designed to serve the working poor, non-AFDC and non-General Assistance low income families. Work with families included assessment of individual needs, development of an action plan to address family needs, and support for families as they worked to meet their goals. In addition to working with families, the project was also designed to improve linkages between self-sufficiency service providers in Anoka County, to identify barriers to self-sufficiency experienced by families, and to advocate for action to address those boundaries.

The project coordinator served as evaluator. The evaluation reports focused on program progress, summaries of intake data, case studies, and discussion of barriers to self-sufficiency.

The program ceased operation in the Spring of 1991. Over three years, 126 families received intake services and 53 requested case management services. The final evaluation reported that most screened families (58%) were ready for some form of job training and did not request case management services; 71% of the families who requested case management services remained involved for three or more meetings. Intensive case management services were provided to 14 families. Staff felt that the clinical perspective provided by staff increased agency sensitivity to mental health issues faced by participants.

Synthesis Trends

Synthesis process. As noted earlier, the purpose of the cluster synthesis was to look across all seven Effective Parenting/Family Stability programs for patterns which cut across outcome claims and implementation experiences. The evaluation team was interested not only in what happens to participants but what claims were made for changes in agencies, communities, and policies as well. More information was needed to fully understand the dynamics and interrelationships among participants, programs, agencies, communities, and policies. Data for the synthesis included project evaluations and was supplemented by site visits, interviews with project directors and staffs, phone conversations, and interviews with community experts. At three intervals summaries of evaluation and interview findings were prepared and discussed with staffs to clarify issues and obtain responses to specific questions. The synthesis process included the development of an impact matrix for each program based on a thorough review of individual program claims, classification of program claims, and assessments of the strength of program claims. Impact matrices for individual projects were then analyzed for crosscutting trends and themes.

The synthesis process was both inductive and exploratory. Two insights from the process are important to share before outcome trends and programming themes are discussed.

First of all, the team found it helpful to distinguish long-term impacts from intermediate outcomes. Long-term impacts for effective parenting/family stability programs, for example, focus on families feeling part of their communities, social and academic success in schools, reduced family violence, and, ultimately, well-functioning, healthy families. For comprehensive FIP programs long-term goals include sustainable economic stability of families, well-functioning healthy families, and staying off welfare and above the poverty line. Many factors beyond the control of programs affect long-term outcomes, for example, the state of the economy, public policies, programs' dependence on funding cycles, demographic trends and general social patterns. Moreover, the longitudinal designs necessary to study long-term effects are expensive, methodologically complex and well beyond the data collection capacities of operating programs.

What this means is that documenting long-term outcomes and impacts is a research task, not a program evaluation function. Attaining long-term outcomes is beyond the exclusive control of these programs; definitively documenting such outcomes is beyond their mission and resources. Thus individual project evaluations and the synthesis appropriately focus on intermediate outcomes.

Second, an important breakthrough came when we understood that the various levels of FIP activity and impact were interrelated. Changes in participants, staff, programs, agencies, policies and the poverty environment are interconnected systemically. There is consistency in the meaning and direction of patterns at these different levels of analysis.

In examining FIP patterns the team found that how people are treated affects how they treat others: responsiveness reinforces responsiveness, flexibility supports individualization and empowerment breeds empowerment. Effective FIP programs emphasized the importance of individualized, responsive and respectful work with families in poverty. But staff cannot (or will not) be individually responsive and supportive in program environments that are rigid and bureaucratic. Staff tend to treat program participants the way they are treated as professionals. If the program administration and environment are rigid, rules-oriented and punitive, the staff will be rigid, rules-oriented and blaming with participants. If the program environment and administration are flexible, responsive, nurturing and supportive, staff in that environment are more likely to interact with participants in ways that are responsive, nurturing and supportive. That's because staff and participants are in a systems relationship. The system includes funders as well. In this case, McKnight worked with programs to be responsive to the actual situations of program participants. Grantees responded by looking for new ways to include rather than exclude and paying attention to variations in need rather than forcing participants into standardized, predetermined program services.

There is one other level of impact in this chain of interconnections; that is the effects of programs on the agencies and systems of which they are a part. McKnight funding gave grantees a certain degree of power, confidence, and autonomy such that grantee programs made demands on host organizations and cooperating units of government to be responsive and flexible. In many cases grantees found that they could not do what needed to be done to assist participants because of agency or government rules and restrictions. Ordinarily programs lack the power or confidence to challenge system barriers to effectiveness. Many FIP programs, however, with the full support of McKnight, formulated strategies to overcome system barriers and thereby create a more flexible and responsive environment for themselves. Even as grantees were often called on to be advocates for families in poverty and help those families become assertive in overcoming system barriers they encountered, so also grantees became assertive in working to change organizational and system barriers to program effectiveness. In some cases, FIP programs changed the agencies in which they were housed, moving those host agencies toward greater flexibility and responsiveness.

Outcome trends. In general, the analysis of intermediate outcomes showed that participants are demonstrating progress on important and measurable outcomes that are critical steps to becoming healthy, stable families and effective parents. Cluster outcome trends are listed in Table 1. A complete discussion of these outcomes is available elsewhere (Mueller, 1993). Discussion of one outcome trend is included to illustrate the relationship between categories of project claims and synthesis trends. Technical summaries were prepared for each project and can be obtained, along with project evaluation reports, from The McKnight Foundation.

Participants took positive steps and demonstrated progress. In all cases, programs document positive steps made by participants which have the *potential* of improving the quality of participants' lives–*over time.* In many cases, the actions taken by participants demonstrate changes in knowledge, practice, and skills. It is important to understand that the concept of participant change is relative–what is significant progress for one family represents a minor modification or change for another. In addition, types of claims vary for different programs. Categories of documented claims are listed below.

- Parents make positive changes in parenting practices. This includes the use of appropriate controls and discipline practices, improved feeding practices and food choices, increased interaction with their children, improved communication with children, and increased monitoring of child care services.

- Adult parents enroll in a range of educational programs and classes. This includes parent education, general education degree (GED), English as a second language (ESL), vocational-technical education, and community college programs. In addition, some adults complete programs and some gain employment.
- Parents demonstrate knowledge of appropriate parenting practices and child development concepts.
- Parents improve problem-solving, planning, and decision-making abilities.
- Children show progress and readiness for Head Start and Kindergarten. This includes greater interest and involvement in toys and educational materials; more appropriate behavior and interaction with other children; comfortable response to other adults.
- Children show fewer school problems.
- Children demonstrate improved ability to attend to task, resolve conflict, and improved social skills.
- Families improve capacity to deal with day-to-day problems. This includes parent motivation for problem-solving; reduced use of physical punishment; family understanding of child care and child development issues; reduction in school problems; established linkages to other family support services. In addition, three months following participation families report improved relations among family members.
- Program families reduce rates of child readmits to emergency shelter. Readmit rates are lower for program families than controls for six month period.

PROGRAMMING THEMES

Site visits, staff interviews, program and evaluation reports provided information about how staff reflect on both implementation experiences and effectiveness. It is important to keep in mind that each program faced unique challenges and opportunities during implementation and each responded in different ways. However, general trends did emerge from the synthesis about factors which

---

TABLE 1

Outcome Trends–Effective Parenting/Family Stability Programs

Individuals and Families

Programs were successful in reaching low income and working poor families. In addition, programs found that the families they worked with were more unique than similar and the issues families faced were more complex than anticipated.

Social isolation was reduced for individuals and families. Programs enhanced participants' informal and formal support networks.

Participants took positive steps and demonstrated progress.

Program and Agency Outcomes

In all programs, staff articulated new understanding of families in poverty and what it takes to provide effective service delivery.

Community Level Outcomes

In addition to providing services to under-served communities, programs influenced how others within communities (professionals, individuals, other programs) think about and approach poverty issues.

Policy Level Outcomes

Programs did not have much impact on public policy, but public policy and policy changes did have significant impact on programs.

---

both support and limit effectiveness. Programming themes are listed in Table 2.

Factors Supporting Effectiveness

Flexibility and responsiveness to participant needs and strengths sets the stage for participant and program change. Families bring to programs unique sets of issues and experiences. To provide effective support, staffs found they must adapt their work to fit the personal circumstances of the families with whom they worked. For

philosophy followed is that when assisting families with complex problems it is important to put exhibited behavior in context; what is maladaptation in one setting may be healthy adaptation in another. The task in complex cases is to bridge realities and assist families through modeling and collaborative problem-solving to deal with problems in their own context.

Clear program boundaries and purposeful flexibility focus action on outcomes. Clarity about a program's purpose and structure allows attention to be focused on maximizing intervention strategies. When the program's mission is clear, staff attention is focused on participants, discovering what can be accomplished and how. Programs with the strongest claims were clear, almost from start-up, about what they wanted to achieve and the outside limits of what could be provided. Within those bounds, these programs remained highly flexible and adapted strategies to meet individual needs despite changes in their operating environment. In the most effective programs a strong sense of mission is the stable core from which flexibility flows. However, flexibility is not an end in itself. Flexibility is a means to the end of effectiveness. A program needs flexibility, the capacity to adapt to changing conditions, to better attain its purposes.

Two examples are helpful here. In one program staff encountered numerous obstacles in helping single parent fathers find housing. Rather than exclude fathers from the program or side step the issue by referring the problem to other agencies, staff remained committed. The search time for finding housing was longer and more contacts were needed to solve the problem. What is important is that the participants' issue was considered to be within the program's mission; the challenge was to solve the problem.

In another case, a program's primary collaborator experienced budget cuts which decreased the level of services the agency could provide in the community. Rather than eliminate screening and assessment services provided by the collaborator, Public Health Nursing, or demanding strict compliance to their agreement, which would have limited the ability of the collaborator to serve other families in the community, Family Resource Center staff assumed responsibility for most of the activity. The staff were clear about their purpose and the role of assessment in supporting their work with families, and the need to be flexible in solving problems.

Effective programs assist families in obtaining basic needs. The capacity of a program to provide effective referrals, follow-through, and ongoing support sets the stage for later work. It facilitates progress. The most effective programs developed extensive contacts, up-to-date operating knowledge of human service and educational systems. Staff distinguished high quality from mediocre human service and educational providers. They developed aggressive follow-through strategies and organizational resources to support both emergency and long-term participant needs. Staffs in the most effective projects were savvy actors in the marketplace of human service and educational providers.

In addition, referral and assistance services were highly integrated into their work. With one exception, the most effective programs did not distinguish referral and assistance support as a separate component or mention it as a factor supporting effectiveness. In other words, the capacity to provide referrals and follow-through is taken for granted. It is basic and integrated into good management.

Effective programs actively seek, manage, and use information. Program staffs with the strongest claims tend to be active information users and seekers. In these cases, knowledge-generating processes were integrated into day-to-day operating practices to a greater extent than in other programs.

The most successful programs are characterized by a high level of information exchange and learning; they used information to adapt strategies and management approaches. Information flow included both systematic and informal channels. Systematic channels are structured and include highly focused program monitoring and evaluation strategies. Informal channels include regular meetings to discuss participant issues and program approaches; relationships with other individuals who have an interest in a participant's progress, e.g., neighbors, teachers, friends; relationships with community groups, agencies, policy decision makers, colleagues in their home agency and other professionals.

All programs had both systematic and informal information channels. However, the most successful ones integrated multiple channels into day-to-day work. They had a diverse range of information sources and the capacity to synthesize and use the information. In the most successful, coordinators played an active role in evaluation design decisions; facilitated both data collection and worker access through on-line systems; supported staff use of these systems; and assisted staff in translating evaluation information for use in their work with families. These coordinators also used evaluation information to assess trends and progress. In addition to integrating systematic information into the work, the most successful coordinators maintained active relationships with participants, colleagues in their home agencies, other community groups and programs. They were active in professional practice networks. The key point here is that coordinators assumed responsibility for information. They made sure information was shared, discussed, and used.

Long-term foundation funding (5 years or more) and commitment to promote effectiveness in programs. Staff from different programs mentioned the importance of foundation support for new ventures for a minimum of 5 years. They also emphasized that funds must be available for evaluation. The shared benefit is better information on program models and outcomes. The pay off for programs is sufficient time for start-up and implementation. Staff specifically noted that evaluation would not be done without foundation support: *"Evaluation was valuable. No question. I'm glad we did it. I'm glad McKnight funded it. But we wouldn't have done it without McKnight funding."*

Professional trust and reciprocal flexibility characterize successful partnerships. Locally based partnerships, in which each partner has an active role in decision-making and service delivery, were important in achieving fast start-up and maintaining ongoing program effectiveness. Resource and policy changes experienced by one or more partners, a common risk of collaborative ventures, effected several projects. In those cases, staffs found that good working relationships and trust were needed to facilitate cooperative adaptation to unanticipated changes.

Thorough training, screening, and professional support are essential for high quality volunteer services to families. Two programs included substantial volunteer components. In The Black Family Parenting Education Program, a train-the-trainer approach was used. Church lay leaders were provided parent education training and served as parent educators. In Family To Family Ties, volunteer families were matched with a low income family and served as a family support partner. The following points summarize key observations from these two programs regarding the use of volunteers.

- High quality training is essential for effective volunteer teaching.
- Professional screening and sensitivity to participant and volunteer needs is important in matching volunteers with participant families. The purpose of screening is to identify families dealing with issues which would overwhelm volunteers and be better served by professionals. In addition, screening volunteers is important to protect participants. Screening is facilitated through individual meetings with volunteers and potential participants. Individual meetings, over a period of time, allow both volunteers and participants to consider their expectations and address concerns before a formal match is made.
- Formalized statement of boundaries guide volunteer-participant relationships. Boundaries for the volunteer/family relationship are established during the first meeting between the volunteer and participant families and formalized in a concrete, written statement.
- Professional staff are needed to support volunteer-participant relationships. Professional staff help volunteers reflect on their evolving relationship, note contributions, and assist with difficult problems. In addition, professional staff push volunteers to move beyond simplistic perceptions of poverty issues and solutions. Staff help volunteers view participant families as peers by identifying shared experiences and common problems.

Factors Limiting Effectiveness

All programs identified barriers which constrained program effectiveness. Projects differed in how barriers were experienced and addressed. For example, programs with the strongest claims identified more external than internal barriers which challenged program effectiveness. In addition, the more effective programs were more aggressive in meeting the challenges.

Competition for funds and demands for innovation strain agency capabilities. Competition for both public and private funds is intense and staying in business is an ongoing challenge for most programs. All staffs discussed concerns about their future work. In many cases, staffs felt that long-term sustainability has more to do with the ability to attract funds than demonstrated effectiveness.

Grantee discussion of this theme emphasized the tendency of both government agencies and foundations to fund "innovative" programs and special interests. This makes it difficult for programs to have a strong, coherent, mission. One FIP director said:

> The politics of funding creates mission chaos and keeps us from building effectiveness over the long term. We keep getting jerked around by short-term political winds. It's hard to stay mission focused when every funder wants your mission to be whatever they are willing to provide money for this week. We use up a lot of energy dealing with mission conflicts imposed from the outside. (Patton, 1992)

External events detract both staff attention and resources from participants. All programs identified external events or changes in their operating context which had the potential of limiting their effectiveness. The following list represents outside factors which had to be addressed during implementation.

- Quality of services and intake policies of other human or educational services.
- Changes in partner capacity.
- Changes in education policy, e.g., mandatory preschool screening of all four-year-olds expected to impact service delivery.
- School level policy changes.
- Funder requirements, e.g., multiple accountabilities and varied specifications.
- Competition, e.g., increase in the number of intensive in-home programs.

- Reduction in shelter placements by county. Decreased funds for shelter placement increased competition for participants among programs. In addition, individuals who were placed tended to have exceptionally severe and complex problems.
- New legislation which recognizes program effectiveness, mandates new service delivery requirements, but provides insufficient funding for program delivery.
- Limited financial resources of Black churches which proved to be a barrier to program continuation.

Demands placed on projects by outside events are common. Most programs face challenges which are beyond their control. The key point is that in responding to challenges resources are diverted and, in many cases, the level of attention focused on participants is reduced.

Staff turnover and the inability to ethnically match staff to participants limits effectiveness. Four programs experienced staffing issues. Problems included: persistent high staff turnover rates, turnover during start-up, insufficient staffing, and low staff turnover. These staffing problems affected the continuity of delivery, the capacity to deliver services, or, in the case of low staff turnover, delayed matching the staff ethnicity to changing neighborhood demographics. Except for one program which identified compensation rates as the source of persistent difficulties, all developed strategies to address their staffing issue.

Ethnically matching staff and participants is an ongoing challenge common to all FIP programs. Minnesota programs for families in poverty commonly bring together predominately middle class, white staff with people of other cultures, especially poor people of color. These cultural differences are barriers. A major issue for FIP programs, largely unresolved, has been dealing with socioeconomic and racial differences between staff and participants.

Limited capacity constrains programs' ability to meet complex needs and new demands. Four programs identified gaps or constraints in their capacity which limited effectiveness. In several cases, the program model was insufficient and additional services were needed; specifically, job training and therapeutic counseling.

Staffs in these programs reported they were not prepared to assist families or individuals with multiple life support issues, personal issues, or those below average in cognitive abilities.

In another case, demand for services by community residents was much higher than anticipated. The project's attempts to meet the demand were complicated when new legislation was passed which required expansion of services but lacked sufficient funding to effectively implement them.

CONCLUSION AND IMPLICATIONS

This report focused on the major outcomes and lessons learned from seven effective parenting/family stability programs. The purpose of these programs was to support families as they took steps to improve the quality of their lives and worked towards getting out of poverty. Staff provided support by working with participants to identify strengths, find assistance for critical needs, improve parenting skills, develop practical strategies, and encourage participants as they take control of their lives. One finding is that the involved families were more unique than similar and the issues they faced were more complex than anticipated. Consequently, approaches, agency policies, and operating practices were modified in order to meet participants' unique needs.

Documented claims show that these programs were successful in reducing social isolation and connecting families to needed services. Families in turn demonstrated improved parenting skills, enhanced knowledge of child development, improved family relationships, and children made improvements in school. In addition, some parents enrolled in educational programs and some found employment.

A major finding was that how people are treated affects how they treat others: responsiveness reinforces responsiveness, flexibility supports individualization and empowerment breeds empowerment. Common themes related to effectiveness included having a clear sense of mission, being responsive to client needs, being flexible in working with diverse clientele, taking a comprehensive, strategic approach and actively seeking and using information.

AUTHOR NOTE

Marsha Mueller's work includes a broad range of evaluation projects; poverty programs; programs for homeless youth; adolescent pregnancy prevention programs; education; cooperative extension; youth development; business and organizational development; judicial education, and alternative school programs. Mueller has authored numerous reports, contributed to professional journals, and taught evaluation classes.

Michael Patton is the author of five major books on evaluation and numerous articles. In addition to directing a consulting business, Dr. Patton serves as a core faculty member for the Union Institute, Cincinnati, OH, and is on the faculty of the Center for Public Policy, Union Institute, Washington, D.C.

REFERENCES

Kagan, S., Powell, D., Weissbourd, B. & Zigler, E. (Eds.) (1987). *America's Family Support Programs*. New Haven: Yale University Press.

Kahn, A., & Kamerman, S.B. (1992, Fall). Integrating Services Integration: A Story Unfolding. *National Center for Children in Poverty News and Issues*, p. 3.

Mueller, M.R. (1992). *The McKnight Foundation Effective Parenting/Family Stability Programs Synthesis Report*. Minneapolis: The McKnight Foundation.

Patton, M.Q. (1992). *The McKnight Foundation Aid to Families in Poverty Initiative Synthesis of Themes, Patterns and Lessons Learned*. Minneapolis: The McKnight Foundation.

Schorr, L.B. (1989). *Within Our Reach*. New York: Doubleday.

The McKnight Foundation. (1991, December). *The McKnight Foundation Aid to Families in Poverty Program, Mid-Point Report*. Minneapolis: The McKnight Foundation.

Weiss, H.B. & Halpern, R. (1990, December). *Community-Based Family Support and Education Programs: Something Old or Something New?* New Haven: Yale University School of Public Health.

Weiss, H.B. & Jacobs, F.H. (Eds.) (1988). *Evaluating Family Programs*. Hawthorn New York: Aldine De Gruyter.

Intervention with Families
in Extreme Distress (FED)

Shlomo A. Sharlin
Michal Shamai

SUMMARY. The FED (Families in Extreme Distress) Project described in this article was developed as an intervention model for families in extreme distress. The concept of "families in extreme distress" includes not only those families which have been widely regarded as "multi-problem families" for decades, but also those which may appear to be like any other middle class family. The disorganization in family functioning that is created by an interaction of many problems results in a durable distress which is repeated throughout successive generations.

The intervention design of this project was structured and short-term, and each family in the group met once a week in their own home for ten sessions with a therapeutic team composed of three workers. The target of the intervention was the functioning of the entire family as a unit; and goals included clarifying boundaries, strengthening roles, and developing a communication system.

Analysis of the therapeutic sessions revealed several techniques which are useful for intervention with the FED population. The intervention process with these families should be multilevel and case management should not only include providing family therapy, but also advocating and mediating with various institutions in the community, as well as making connections for financial assistance.

Shlomo A. Sharlin is Director, The Center for Research of Study of the Family, School of Social Work, University of Haifa, Haifa, Israel. Michal Shamai is Director, Regional Center for Instruction and Family Therapy, Haifa, Israel.

[Haworth co-indexing entry note]: "Intervention with Families in Extreme Distress (FED)." Sharlin, Shlomo A., and Michal Shamai. Co-published simultaneously in *Marriage & Family Review* (The Haworth Press, Inc.) Vol. 21, No. 1/2, 1995, pp. 91-122; and: *Exemplary Social Intervention Programs for Members and Their Families* (ed: David Guttmann, and Marvin B. Sussman) The Haworth Press, Inc., 1995, pp. 91-122. Multiple copies of this article/chapter may be purchased from The Haworth Document Delivery Center [1-800-3-HAWORTH; 9:00 a.m. - 5:00 p.m. (EST)].

91

While some major policy changes may be required to meet the financial and manpower needs involved in such a model, this demonstration project indicates that investing the right resources is worthwhile for effecting change within the FED population.

REVIEW OF LITERATURE

Much of the literature concerning the study of multiproblem families has tried to explain and understand the reasons why such families are created as well as the factors behind their continued existence. This phenomenon was extensively researched from the end of the 1940s through the 1970s. After World War II, during which the concern for the very existence of humanity was of utmost importance, an era of concern began for social interest and the quality of life.

The term "multiproblem families," which was widely used during this period, referred primarily to lower class families who suffered from poverty and other interpersonal problems. These families were characterized by poor verbal ability, physical appearance and health status, as well as poor living conditions. The interaction between their different problems created a disorganized family structure accompanied by difficulties in parenting and marital relationships and antisocial behavior. Such families could thus be easily identified through observation.

From the early studies (Lewis, 1959; Gans, 1962), it became clear that the phenomenon of multiproblem families is not a consequence of economic hardship alone. More and more scholars began speaking of such concepts as "personal and social disorganization" (Geismar & La Sorte, 1964), "poverty personality" (Harrington, 1962), and "poverty culture" (Lewis, 1961). The basic argument was that in order to reach such a level of dysfunction in so many areas, there must be additional variables which serve to maintain the extreme distress and preserve it throughout several generations.

These successive generations repeat the cycle of the "poverty culture" with children adopting the "poverty personality" in their emotional development and socialization. Individuals born into disorganized families are exposed to a world which created emotional and behavioral difficulties. These are expressed by acting out, low level of frustration, impulsivity, lack of capacity for self-control, low level of verbal ability, difficulty in abstract thinking, and identity problems (Bernstein, Jeremy & Marcus, 1986). Children have numerous difficulties in adjusting to school. Many drop out at an early age and participate in antisocial activities, such as delinquency, drug and alcohol abuse in order to provide stimulation to their leisure time (Malone, 1963; Gans, 1963; Deutsch, 1963). The way of life of the poverty culture increases the tendencies towards disease, mental illness and antisocial behavior (Harrington, 1962).

Polansky et al. (1970; 1971; 1972a; 1972b; 1981) conducted a series of longitudinal studies in the 1970s which focused on mothers who neglect their children. Several types of women were identified who are likely to be encountered in treating a neglect situation. Polansky and his associates were particularly interested in the type of women fitting the "apathy-futility syndrome." These were women who appeared to be passive, withdrawn, and lacking in expression, suggesting that the disability largely resided within. Their living in poverty made it more difficult for them to cope and resulted in severe child neglect. Their children suffered from extreme physical and emotional deprivation, intellectual deficiency, and character disorders.

An attempt to define the characteristics of multiproblem families in a psychiatric context was done by Dax and Haggar (1977). They assert that the standard psychiatric nomenclature, such as "schizophrenia," "borderline," "psychotic," etc., are irrelevant and do not contain the problematic complexity of distress families. To develop an intervention according to psychiatric definitions is not relevant, since it does not include all the characteristics of these populations. Dax and Haggar (1977) argue that the nature of problems presented by multiproblem families is such that it would be better to describe them not specifically, but rather, in general terms. Therefore, a much better way to define and identify multiproblem families would be to describe their characteristics.

Defining Families in Extreme Distress (FED)

We prefer to use the term Families in Extreme Distress, or FED, rather than the term "multiproblem families" which has been widely used over the last few decades. The concept of Families in

Extreme Distress includes the group of multiproblem families, but also relates to families that may appear to be like any other middle-class family. Such families have adopted middle-class standards of housing and physical appearance; yet, their family functioning is similar to that of multiproblem families. Although this group has succeeded in improving their verbal skills, housing conditions, and even financial situation, they have not managed to overcome the values and habits that characterize lower-class multiproblem families. This group often misleads social workers to try to treat them with approaches and techniques relevant to middle-class populations.

Behind this middle-class facade, we find an interaction between at least five problems which creates disorganized functioning within the families. We define FED as families who are characterized by at least five of these different facets: (1) poverty; (2) poor housing conditions; (3) troubled marital relationship; (4) multiple children; (5) difficulties in parenting; (6) lack of support systems; (7) antisocial activities; (8) substance abuse; and (9) poor physical and mental health status. The subsequent disorganization created by this interaction leads to a durable distress; hence, we term it as families in extreme distress (FED). In such families, the only organized and stable state is their disorganization, lack of stability, and inconsistent habit patterns.

Intervention with Multiproblem Families

There is a diversity of experience in treating multiproblem families. Some approaches have emphasized programs on the community level, such as those in schools, neighborhoods, or community centers. Others have centered more on the belief that the family is a social unit which must be the focus of intervention if norms and values are to be changed (Spiegel, 1959; Riesman, 1962, 1973).

The literature that deals with treating multiproblem families emphasizes how difficult it is to work with them. Lorion (1978) provides us with two explanations as to why such interventions result in little success: (1) the way human service workers relate to the poor population in distress; (2) the way the population in distress relates to treatment.

Many workers were found to relate negatively to the multiproblem families, and expressed themselves in such a manner that one would question their ability to deal with the therapeutic processes underlying problem-solving (Schneiderman, 1965). In studies which investigated workers' relationships to distress clients, it was doubtful if these individuals could be helped for the following reasons: (a) the workers feeling ill-at-ease with such clients; (b) the stereotypic perceptions of workers regarding their clients; and (c) the perceptions of some workers that their work with these clients was a waste of time (Baum et al., 1966; Kaplan et al., 1968). How the worker relates to clients influences expectations of the outcome, the worker's empathic abilities, and her or his motivation to succeed. Such variables were found to correlate positively with treatment outcomes (Parloff, Waskow & Wolf, 1978).

Other studies attempted to view variables that characterized how the multiproblem population felt about treatment intervention. Lorion (1978) points out that studies conducted in the 1950s showed negative relationships, and the lack of belief that multiproblem families had in intervention and its chance of succeeding. Other studies also confirmed that clients did not know what to expect from the treatment (Hollingshead & Redlich, 1958). Studies of the 1960s and 1970s showed that the gap between the middle-class and lower-class populations, which were described as multiproblem families or disadvantaged families, became smaller in relation to expected outcomes of treatment. The expectation which multiproblem families had from intervention was that the worker should be active and supportive (Aronson & Overall, 1966).

Another variable studied in relation to multiproblem populations is the degree of fitness between the treatment approach and the family. Most studies indicate that intervention models which use dynamic oriented psychotherapy are not useful with multiproblem families. However, a few studies describe attempts made by workers who utilized dynamic oriented psychotherapy. These studies underline the importance of the therapist in being flexible when providing support, acceptance, protection, and direct advice. Thus, clients' motivation and capacity towards treatment increased and resulted in changes in reality perception, capacity for emotional control, and the ability for joining inner processes. As stated, the therapists' flexibility and democracy provided the major components for change (Gould, 1967; Lerner, 1972).

Short-term intervention and behavioral approaches are more commonly used in treating multiproblem populations. This is due to the nature of the treatment, which focuses on the symptoms and is limited to a particular time frame. Lorion (1978) points out that very few studies have been done on short-term intervention and its effectiveness with such populations. Some studies have indicated that multiproblem populations benefit from short-term treatment (Yamamato & Goin, 1966; Koegler & Brill, 1967; Crosthers, 1972); however, these studies relate only to the advantage of the worker using focused treatment and not to the specific advantage for the multiproblem population.

Experts on multiproblem families have indicated that family therapy may be the optimal intervention for dealing with a poverty culture and the poverty personality which develops and is preserved in the chaotic family (Gans, 1962; Miller, 1964; Giordano, 1973). Family therapy, as opposed to individual therapy, enables one to overcome the myth that multiproblem populations are untreatable (Salig, 1976).

Since the 1960s, several attempts have been made in treating poor and multiproblem families, some combining community work with family therapy. Mannino and Shore (1972) report on a program that aimed to teach multiproblem families how to communicate with relevant institutions in the community, such as schools, Departments of Social Services, or medical services. The purpose of their program was to promote the effectiveness of these families in making use of available services and to change the structure and functioning of the family.

The work of Minuchin and associates (1967; 1974) has served as an inspiration to many who work with multiproblem families. Their treatment involves changing the structure of the family, which they believe will result in improved functioning. Simultaneously, they create new boundaries between parents and children by empowering parents to act appropriately in the roles. Minuchin's work was further developed by his followers, and in the 1970s and 1980s, Aponte reports on a few attempts of coping with multiproblem families (1974; 1976a; 1976b; 1979; 1986). Gurman (1973) and

Beck (1976), in analyzing the outcome of family treatment with multiproblem families in the U.S., report on significant improvement as a result of intervention and willingness of the population both to cope and to join the treatment.

Nevertheless, most writers emphasize that there is a need for a set of different approaches in order to reach multiproblem families and cope with problems which have already existed for several generations. The principles suggested in the literature for treating multiproblem families include: (a) reaching out and conducting the treatment at home (Rabin et al., 1982); (b) employing crisis intervention while cooperating with the mental health system and the Department of Social Services, in conjunction with vigorous action by the social worker (Argyles & MacKenzie, 1970); (c) utilizing the social worker's ties with the community to overcome resistance and anger that exists between the family and institutions in the community; (d) using focused intervention which aims to achieve one clear goal during a limited time period, usually between 8-16 meetings (Reid, 1985); (e) using creative techniques, such as family painting, arts and crafts, storytelling during treatment, etc., while the therapist takes on leadership and parental roles; (f) using specific concepts, such as Verbal Accessibility (V.A.) (Polansky, 1971; Wells, 1981), in which the abilities to effectively express emotions and solve problems are considered as an integral part of family communication and functioning; (g) developing a preventive program for young children (Hardy & MacMahon, 1981; Tomlinson & Peters, 1981; Starkie, 1984; Heying, 1985; Bernstein et al., 1986).

In general, social service interventions are suitable for the treatment of multiproblem families (Coulshed, 1983; Jenkins, 1983; Hardy & MacMahon, 1981). However, in order to implement such a program successfully, it is necessary to focus first on reducing the anger, suspicion and hate which these families have towards social service workers, as well as the antipathies of professionals towards such families (Weitzman, 1985; Aponte, 1986; Schlosberg & Kagan, 1988).

In particular, emigrating families are one population known to suffer from extreme distress (Minuchin et al., 1967). The sample used in the following project is composed largely of families who have emigrated to the State of Israel, many of whom have experienced a change from a traditional or religious culture to a secular one. Such marked transitions can serve as fertile ground for the creation of distressed families.

Families in Extreme Distress (FED) Project

The FED Project described here is an effort developed by The Center for the Study and Research of the Family, at the University of Haifa, in collaboration with the Haifa Center for Training and Family Therapy for the Ministry of Labor and Social Affairs. The project was developed in collaboration with and for the Department of Social Services (DSS) to experiment with an intervention model for families in extreme distress. The project was designed to be carried out in two communities, and a FED Center was planned for each DSS. The project goals were as follows:

1. To undertake an innovative demonstration project with families regarded as FED.
2. To find suitable intervention methods for bringing about a defined change.
3. To intervene in order to change the present situation.
4. To integrate intervention systems and resources so as to induce a planned change.
5. To develop a working model for intervention, such as a FED Center in a Department of Social Services.

A schematic description of the project structure is seen in Figure 1. The major strategy was to form an intervention team composed of three workers with different roles as follows:

1. An expert Family Therapist (F.T.) who serves as the team leader and is in charge of conducting the therapy with the family.
2. A social worker from the DSS who is the permanent worker assigned to the participating family and who serves as a Case Manager (C.M.). The worker's role is to link the family with community institutions and provide continuity of care after the project is over.
3. A social work aide, usually a second year MSW student, who serves as a Project Coordinator (P.C.). The P.C. arranges for meetings and therapy sessions and assumes a co-therapist's role when needed, and provides feedback to the team.

FIGURE 1. FED Center

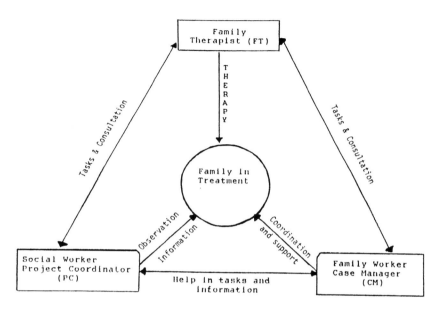

Sample

Twenty families were selected from two participating communities, with each DSS providing ten of the "most difficult families" on their rosters. The average FED family was composed of a husband, 40 years old, and a wife, 34 years old. Seventy-five percent of husbands and wives were of North-African origin. Most of their lives were spent in Israel, having emigrated between the ages of four and six. They were from a traditional religious sect, and their education was at a 7-8th grade level. Fifty percent of the husbands did not perform their compulsory military service, and none of the women served. (In Israel, women are obligated to serve in the armed forces for two years unless exempted on religious grounds.)

The majority of the couples were from second generation FED families (75%). Most of them had debts, and half of them were unemployed. Fifty percent were diagnosed as having physical or mental health problems. The couples had lived together for 15 years and, on average, had six children. Half of the couples married because the wife was pregnant out of wedlock or because they were forced into marriage by their families. All the couples had several periods of separation after which they returned to each other.

Intervention Goals

The goals of the intervention techniques were: strengthening the couple's family system by clarifying boundaries; developing a communication system; strengthening parental and child roles; and, where appropriate, suggesting new roles for the husband and other family members. In each family, we chose to focus on one or two of these goals in a short-term intervention approach. We also recognized the need among the social workers (Case Managers) to change their perceptions of their role in order to prevent the development of a "coalition of despair" between the workers and the FED families (Shamai, 1989).

Intervention Procedure

Each family in the group met once a week for ten one-hour sessions with the team in their home. All sessions were recorded in order to study the process. The Haifa Center for Training and Family Therapy provided ongoing supervision of the F.T.s at least once every two weeks and, if needed, more frequently. Once a month, the entire FED project staff met for a teaching and training day. During these days, workers reported on their contacts with the families, presented case conferences, and raised specific issues. Treatment sessions were evaluated as well as planned for the future.

A Multi-Professional Team (M.P.T.) was organized by the C.M. to join the FED intervention team for briefing and coordination treatment efforts. Members of the M.P.T. are professionals in the community with whom the family interacts, such as the family physician, nurse, teacher, school headmaster, lawyer, etc. The specific composition of each team varies according to the needs of the family and the outcome of intervention. The team, directed by the P.C. and supervised by the Project Director, is responsible for sharing information relevant to the family's problems, prioritizing needs, and mediation on behalf of the family with community agencies (see Figure 2).

FIGURE 2. Logistics of the Project

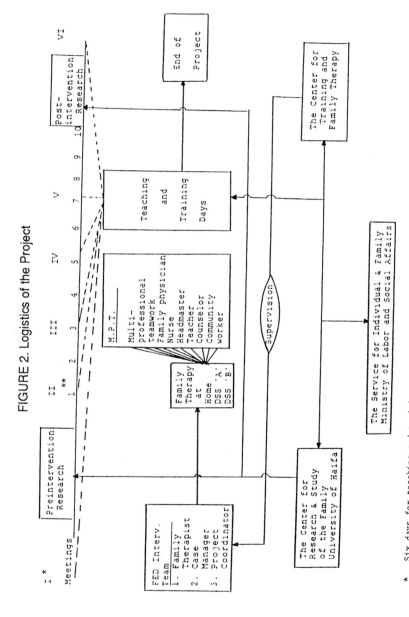

* Six days for teaching and training.

** Ten sessions of intervention with each family.

101

Set of Useful Techniques: "The Tool Box"

Clinical observation and analysis of the therapeutic sessions revealed several techniques which seemed to be useful for intervention with the FED population. Many of these techniques are often used by family therapists, but in order to implement them with the FED families, some accommodations must be made. The techniques include: (1) joining and rejoining with the family; (2) using multilevel intervention; (3) creating boundary systems; (4) using concrete signals; (5) focusing on direct and clear communication; (6) using suggestive techniques; and (7) using creative nonverbal techniques, such as those drawn from art therapy.

1. *Joining and Rejoining with the Family.* Joining with the family is a basic condition for creating and maintaining the therapeutic system (Minuchin & Fishman, 1981). Joining is usually carried out at the beginning of the therapeutic process and allows the family therapist to enter and understand the family's world. As the intervention proceeds, joining becomes a natural part of the therapeutic process. However, with FED families, one cannot take for granted that joining early in the process will suffice. Many families were suspicious of the therapists even at the fifth or sixth meeting. The families were constantly testing the therapists to find out whether they could be trusted. As a result, the therapeutic team had to invest a lot of time and energy during the interventions to rejoin with the families, thereby renewing the commitment of the families to the therapy.

It is known that FED families challenge their therapists by resisting in different ways. Resistance can be explained by the anger and suspicions of the FED population towards the helping professions, especially towards social workers. The previous experience of the families had often involved painful relationships with the helping professions, which had been terminated either by failure or by the therapist's abandonment of the family (Schlosberg & Kagan, 1988). In contrast to middle-class populations, with whom the frame of the therapeutic contract has to be kept in order to increase the effectiveness of the intervention (Mallucio & Marlow, 1974; Seabury, 1976; Fischer, 1978; Shamai, 1987), interventions with the FED population have to focus on the different possibilities of joining and rejoining with the family even if this violates the therapeutic contract.

Case Illustration: Mrs. Shetef expressed a great amount of resistance to the therapeutic intervention. Although she played a significant part in the first three sessions and her desire that Mr. Shetef would return to sleep with her in the same bed was fulfilled, nonetheless her resistance did not decrease. It seemed to the team that Mrs. Shetef was afraid to lose the social worker who was perceived by her as belonging only to her and not to the entire family. When the team arrived at the fourth session at 8:30 a.m., as was planned, they met Mrs. Shetef at the entrance of her house while taking her daughter to the kindergarten. Mrs. Shetef's appearance was unkempt; she was still in her night dress and had not combed her hair. Mrs. Shetef completely ignored the therapeutic team. Then the family therapist approached Mrs. Shetef and told her that she understood the family had just woken up. Mrs. Shetef answered angrily that it was true. The family therapist added that she understood the difficulty in getting up straight for treatment, and suggested that the team would wait a while until the family could get organized or could postpone the meeting until the afternoon. Mrs. Shetef's eyes lit up and she asked the team to wait a few minutes until the family organized itself. The relationship between her and the team was different in this meeting. Mrs. Shetef was more cooperative and expressed less resistance. It seemed that the accepting and caring behavior of the team, as well as the respectful attitude the team had towards her way of organizing time, resulted in changing her behavior.

2. *Using Multilevel Intervention.* Multilevel intervention focuses on the behavioral and emotional functioning of the family, as well as on the level of financial difficulty and the disconnection of the family with social institutions in the community. All of these issues were addressed by the therapeutic team, and such multilevel intervention was accomplished through clear and discrete role definition of each team member. The F.T. was responsible for carrying out the behavioral and emotional interventions; the C.M. was responsible for making the connections with other social institutions; and the P.C. was responsible for serving as a participant observer.

Case Illustration: The Shahars arrived at the fifth meeting expressing anxiety. They talked about their debt and about the large
expenses that could not be controlled. The therapeutic team,
together with the family, decided that the social worker would
meet with the family during the week in order to summarize
the incomes and expenses of the family. At the following
session, the social worker and the family discussed alternative
ways for coping with the financial situation. During the discussion, the family therapist helped to define the role of Mr.
Shahar and Mrs. Shahar in their efforts to improve their financial situation. Special attention was paid to the mutual support
given by each spouse to the other.

It is important to indicate that the different roles of the team
members did not prevent them from acting as co-therapists whenever the family therapist found it necessary. As co-therapists, the team
members discussed and negotiated between themselves in front of
the family. This negotiation not only exposed the family to different
ways of thinking and problem-solving, but sometimes the opposing
assessments in the team put the family in a paradoxical situation
that challenged their motivation to create a solution. It was also
possible that by joining with at least one of the ideas that were
expressed by the team, the resistance of the family members was
lowered (Tomm, 1984; Boscolo et al., 1987). Negotiating in front of
negotiation and problem-solving in which each family member
could listen to the ideas of the others and respond in a respectful
way without recourse to physical violence or psychological abuse.

Case Illustration: During the meetings with the Lev family, Mr. Lev
expressed his anger towards his teenage daughter because she
shaved her legs. When Mr. Lev was asked how he knew this,
he said that his daughter had told his wife, and she had let him
know about it. The therapist, who was a woman and a mother
of two teenage girls, turned to another member in the team,
who was a father of two teenage girls, and asked whether he,
as a father, was used to intervening in feminine matters in his
family. The therapist added that in her family, feminine issues
were her responsibility. The male therapist answered from his
parental position that in his family, the teenage girls usually

turned to his wife with feminine matters. If his wife chose to share some of the issues with him, he listened and expressed his point of view. However, it was clear that his responsibility was to reinforce the trust the girls had in their mother and to let his wife handle it. The female therapist challenged Mr. Lev to control himself in the future if his wife tells him something about their teenage daughter.

3. *Creating a Boundary System.* Disorganization is recognized as the main characteristic of multiproblem families (Pavenstedt, 1965; Minuchin et al., 1967). Creating some organization and defining boundaries, roles and relationships within the family, as well as between the family and society, are among the main goals of family treatment with this population. The project allowed direct and indirect intervention on the issue of organization and boundaries. The structure of the project created a time limit and clearly defined the roles of each team member, with each member assigned specific therapeutic responsibilities. As a result, the intervention had a basic organized framework. Meeting the families in their own homes helped the group to organize and arrive at the meetings on time. We assumed that if families were asked to arrive at the Social Services Department, many of them would not be able to cope with this request.

During treatment, the family therapist worked directly on creating a boundary system by defining rules for the meetings, such as when and how one can speak, or by giving tasks to be accomplished during or between the therapeutic meetings. The therapist used concrete and simple terms in order to explain these rules and tasks. Thus, everyone in the family was able to clearly define his or her role.

Case Illustration: Two teenage girls in the Lev family were deeply enmeshed in their parents' relationship. The girls accepted responsibility for judging their parents' fights and arguments. The family therapist explained to the girls that the arguments and the fights between their parents were the way their parents knew how to communicate. The therapist added that when one of the girls intervened between the parents, she prevented direct communication between her mother and father without being aware of it. This explanation decreased the fear the girls felt whenever their parents began to argue. In addition, the girls were asked to let their parents know that they were aware that a fight was going on by holding up a signal that looked like a green light and then leave the room, thus allowing their parents to make their own decision as to whether or not they wanted to continue the fight.

4. *Using Concrete Signals.* It is clear from previous cases that the therapist had to use concrete signals during the intervention in order to overcome the difficulties which many of the FED families had in understanding and relating to the content of abstract material. The family therapist had to be very creative in order to explain rules and situations whenever the family could not respond to abstract material presented during treatment.

Case Illustration: The Lev family includes twelve members. When the team came to the first meeting, it was impossible to overcome the chaotic behavior of the family and even to get to know each member of the family personally. There was complete disorganization in the room; none of the family members let another talk without intervening, children went in and out of the room constantly, and Mr. and Mrs. Lev argued all the time. After twenty minutes, the family therapist took out two signals that look like traffic lights. One of the signals explained a rule according to which the family would behave during the meeting: only the member who had the green traffic light could speak; for all other members the traffic light was red, which meant "stop" or "be quiet." All the family members understood the rule, since it was taken from everyday life, and they responded to it. In another session with the family, the therapist did not have the traffic light signals with her, so she took from the table two different kinds of fruits, a banana and an orange, as concrete signals for permission to talk.

5. *Focusing on Direct and Clear Communication Within the Family.* Low verbal communication often characterizes multiproblem, or FED, families (Polansky et al., 1970; 1971; 1972a; 1972b). It is important to indicate that communication does exist in FED

families, but the communication is usually nondirect, consists of double messages, and is expressed through violent terms, verbal or physical. The shortage of communication skills prevents direct and clear communication between family members. In working on issues of communication, the family therapist was able to shape communicative skills by reinforcing verbal, direct, and clear messages while suppressing communication which amplified violence and alienation. Techniques like modeling and role-playing followed by intensive support from the therapist were used in building communication skills.

Case Illustration: The Zen family looked for a way to convince their son, Lavee, to go back to school. Lavee had been absent from school for almost three months.

Family Therapist: As we decided in our last meeting, we would try today to help Lavee to return to school. Since all the family members know what school is, and some of the members have also experienced situations of missing school, it is important that all of you are here. (To the father): I think that you, as the father of the family, should open the discussion. I would like to ask you to turn to Lavee and ask him about his difficulties in going back to school.

Father (to the therapist): The problem is that Lavee is very young and not a smart boy. He tries to imitate his brother Alon (who dropped out of school). I tried to explain to him in a nice way, I beat him, and nothing helped.

Therapist (to the father): School is sometimes a very frightening place for young children. (To the other children in the family): What do you think, is it difficult in school?

The other children in the family joined the family therapist and said that it was very difficult in school with their studies, teachers, and friends.

Lavee: Once I even cried in school because I did not have a friend.

Therapist (returning to the father): Please talk with him. Ask him about his difficulties in school.

Father (to the therapist): I know what's difficult for him.

Therapist: Please try, if only for our discussion. You can ask, 'Lavee, what is difficult for you in school?' (Here the therapist
acted as a model.)
Father (to the therapist): Please, leave it. I have already talked with
him. There is nothing more to do.
Therapist: I know that it is very hard to speak with a young child.
But I am sure that even young children have an opinion.
Would you like to try and find out whether your child has an
opinion? (The therapist tried to challenge the father to talk
directly with his son.)
Father: Lavee, what's so hard for you in school?
Lavee: I am embarrassed to go to the new school.
Father: Would you rather go back to your old school?

This was the basis for opening a direct discussion between the
father and his son. The therapist gave an enormous amount of
support to the father, as well as verbal reinforcement, for his good
will in trying to understand Lavee. As the session continued, the
father tried to explain the reasons for Lavee's embarrassment.

Therapist: So, Lavee is embarrassed. (To Lavee): Who in your
family is a specialist in embarrassment?
Lavee: Gilad (his brother, sixteen years old and a very quiet boy).
Gilad: (smiled).
Therapist (to Lavee): If Gilad is the specialist in getting embarrassed, please consult with him on how to get along in the new
school. You are right about being embarrassed in a new place,
and it is very important to know how to get along with a
feeling of embarrassment. Since Gilad is a specialist in embarrassment, he is the one to consult with.
Lavee: (Quiet, does not answer).
Father: Answer her already (rushing him).
Therapist: (to the father): Please, don't rush him. It is very difficult
to know how to ask directly. (The therapist identified with the
father's difficulty, while at the same time she gave a clear
boundary to the father as well as a model for how the father
could understand his children and respect them.) (To Lavee):
Gilad is the one who knows best in your family how to be
embarrassed, and he is the one to talk with about embarrass-

ment. You can't consult with someone who doesn't know how to be embarrassed and live with it.

Lavee (to Gilad): How can I live with it?

Gilad: (Quiet, does not answer).

Father: Answer him . . .

Gilad (to the therapist): He doesn't have to be embarrassed. All his friends are in school.

Therapist (to Gilad): Please, don't talk to me, talk directly to Lavee, like one man to another. Tell him: Don't be embarrassed. You have friends there . . .

Gilad (to Lavee): Don't be embarrassed in school. All your friends are there.

Lavee: But I am embarrassed.

Gilad: By whom?

Lavee: By the new teacher.

Gilad: But there are many friends from the neighborhood and from the club in school.

Lavee: It's the new teacher and the new friends, and lots of friends I used to meet in the club aren't coming to the club anymore.

Gilad: Well, it will take time, but you will get used to the teacher and to the friends. First of all, try to get along with those that you already know and only later with new friends.

Since the family therapist persisted so and would not give up during this session, the family members finally succeeded in communicating directly.

6. *Using Suggestive Techniques.* Suggestive techniques relate to the process of bringing an idea into the mind through association with other ideas that are meaningful to the individual or the family. The use of suggestive techniques has been an integral part of therapeutic interventions without relating to these techniques directly or explicitly. Since the growing interest in Milton Erickson's work and the increasing use of hypnotherapeutic techniques, emphasis has also been placed on the use of suggestive techniques in the therapeutic process.

The influence of suggestivity appears in the literature in two areas. The first area focuses on the influence of suggestivity on the results of treatment, with special attention given to studying the placebo effect in different populations. Many studies show that positive change can occur without giving treatment, but rather, by building up a set of expectations that something–not necessarily therapy–will help (Shapiro & Morris, 1978). According to many studies, it seems that about 33% of the positive results of treatment are related to the placebo effect which is created by the expectations of clients (Bergin & Lambert, 1978). If so, building an expectation system at the beginning of the intervention ought to be an integral and important part when clients are being prepared for therapy.

In the project, special attention was given to creating an expectation system that would provide the FED families with a source of hope for positive change, as well as trust in the skills and experience of the therapeutic team. When the social workers told the families about the project, they presented it as a very special project that would be done together with the University of Haifa. The family therapists who were assigned to the group were introduced as very experienced therapists. The families who were chosen to take part in the project were described as very special families who had been chosen by their social workers in the belief that they could benefit from treatment and improve their functioning. This kind of introduction created a basis for developing a positive expectation system within the families and the social workers who took part in the project. Since we were aware of the relationship between treatment results and therapists' perceived prognosis (Garfield, 1978), it was important to focus on building up positive expectations among the social workers who had many doubts about the ability of the families to change.

The other area of suggestivity relates to messages presented by the therapist to the families or individuals during treatment. These are usually verbal messages connected with the clients' imaginative and semantic representational systems at both the conscious and unconscious levels. These messages are perceived on the conscious level of the client, which sometimes is called the "representational system," as well as on an unconscious level, called the "reference system." The integration between the representational system and the reference system affects the "lead system." The lead system is used by human beings in order to decide whether to accept conveyed information and how to make use of it (Bandler & Grinder, 1979).

In analyzing the therapeutic sessions in the project, it was obvious that the family therapists used many suggestive messages. The suggestive messages were often used to join the families and helped to create some changes in the attitudes and behaviors of the FED families.

Case Illustration: The Levs were ambivalent about joining the project. Their ambivalence was rooted in a fear that the team would support their teenage daughter, Sarah, who wanted to leave home and go to boarding school or to a foster family. The Levs had eleven children; the oldest one had died when she was seven years old after a severe illness, and four of the other ten children were in foster families and boarding schools. The parents had a strong feeling of failure in educating their children.

At the beginning of the treatment, they insisted that one of their daughters, Morit, should come back home from her aunt who functioned as a foster parent for her. The family therapist reduced the anxiety of the Levs and joined with them by using a suggestive message: "You are good parents. You are the kind of parents who see what's good for your children. You will do what's good for your children even if it is very difficult for you, and that means you are good parents." This message was accepted by the parents, since it was related to the family perception of "good" and "bad" in parenting. This message helped the Levs to accept the fact that Morit's leaving her aunt's home would lead to a further crisis. When they perceived themselves as good parents, they dealt with the issue from a position of power and not from a position of failure and weakness. The suggestive message also affected the relationship between Sarah and her parents. She began to perceive them as caring parents. By the end of treatment, Sarah no longer asked to leave home. She described changes at home, especially in the way her parents functioned. It seems that the suggestive message given to the Levs that they were good parents affected not only them, but also their children.

In the last meeting, the team gave each family a written message. These messages included some suggestive elements that connected the therapeutic process with the reality and meaningful aspects of the family. The message was structured so that the representational and the reference systems of the family members would be affected in a way which would challenge the lead system to act towards change.

Case Illustration: This written message was given to the Sahars by the team at the last meeting:

Dear S. (Mrs. S.) and C. (Mr. S.),
It seems to us that after ten meetings, we can summarize and evaluate part of the treatment and find out what was learned during the process that can be available and useful to you in everyday life. In our meetings we focused on your family and your relationship. We realized very easily that the main theme in your relationship is love. Each of you has strong feelings towards the other, both of you trust each other. The love and the trust were built through the years of being together. C., your love to S. is expressed by your appreciation of her and recognition of her honesty, her dedication, and her tendency to have a pessimistic view of life. S., your love to C. is expressed by your appreciation of his honesty, loyalty, dedication, sense of humor, and optimistic ideas. Your love is your strength. You are very strong. You have the strength to build together, and you have the strength to destroy together. (Repeating the word 'strength' many times is a suggestive technique.)
  Through your love, you have built many things in your relationship: you overcame the difficulties in getting pregnant; you overcame the difficulties during the pregnancy; you are trying to cope with the three babies and the financial difficulties, and trying to support each other during the time C. has tried to stop drinking. Both of you admit that you could cope with all the difficulties through mutual support. But with your strength, you also have the ability to destroy. When your relationship begins to deteriorate, you are like a driver who loses the brakes of his car in the middle of a mountain slope. (Since

Mr. S. is the driver, this metaphor is used for a suggestive goal.) Then you are crossing the red line by blaming and humiliating each other, and even by using physical violence. Sometimes it seems that you have not yet found the way to feel your love during the routine of everyday life. You need the excitement, the high volume, and then you either love or hate each other.

What worries us is that in this situation, you lose the loyalty to each other and become loyal to the 'institution of marriage.' The loyalty to the institution of marriage weakens your relationship. When both of you choose to become loyal to the institution of marriage, C. is loyal to his family of origin and S. is loyal to her family of origin. The values of your family, C., required the wife to act according to her husband's demands. The wife must always be loyal and respectful to her husband without raising doubts or questions. In the family of S., intimacy did not exist, and secrets were told without regard for boundaries. In your family, S., you have learned that the woman is always a victim of her husband and that the man is the one to blame for it. Keeping these values of the families of origin prevent you from building your family as a 'common business.' Only when you decide to choose, either in building or in destroying, will you be able to commit yourself to the choice. You have developed a special skill to hurt each other, and in so doing, you also hurt yourselves. When C. is hurt, he usually turns to the bottle and drinking. He then becomes soft, without boundaries and without 'brakes' (here again relating to C.'s world). When S. is hurt, she usually gets an asthma attack, she does not have enough air, her body becomes tense and rigid, and she becomes the 'brakes' (relating to meaningful things in the family).

But, each one of you also has special skills in being dedicated and committed. S. is committed to the housework and to educating and caring for the children. C. is obligated to his job. We think that it is the right time for each of you to invest in your growth. If you do it, then you, C., would be able to learn from S. about how to be sometimes tough like a 'fimo' (a slang term that was used as a metaphor), and S. would have the chance to learn from C. about how to be sometimes soft like play-dough. In both of you we can find the toughness and the softness. We, the team, trust your experience in being committed to each other. If you choose to use this commitment, you will have many chances to complement each other and to use the phrase you often used during treatment: 'you were great.'

7. *Using Creative Nonverbal Techniques.* The use of creative tools has become an integral part of psychosocial therapeutic approaches. Psychodrama, art therapy, bibliotherapy, dance therapy, etc., increase the possibilities of therapeutic interventions we use for different kinds of populations. Many social workers and family therapists integrated aspects of various art approaches into their therapeutic interventions. Integration of techniques that utilize artistic aspects has been common in the area of family therapy for many years. Nonverbal techniques help therapists to overcome the obstacles of low verbal communication ability as well as to increase the intensity of feeling within families that use words as a means of defense and resistance.

Case Illustration: During the first meeting with the Abrahams, the family therapist and the team learned that the family was very ambivalent about taking part in the project. In fact, they joined the project because they had thought they would receive more financial help. As a result, the family therapist was not surprised that the Abrahams were not so enthusiastic about being open in the meeting. Besides being ambivalent about the project, the Abrahams had been described as a closed family, maintaining minimal ties with their extended family and the community. During the meeting, the members of the family hardly talked among themselves. As for the structure of the family, it seemed that the father, Mr. Abraham, was very lonely. The children were with their mother, Mrs. Abraham, who fiercely held on to her status and power.

According to these observations, the therapist decided to reduce the resistance to the intervention while strengthening communication among family members, including the father. At the next meeting, the family therapist brought with her magazines with many pictures. She asked the family to create one family collage from the pictures in the magazines. While the family members created the collage, they asked the family therapist questions. The therapist referred some of the questions to the father in order to encourage verbal communication between the father and the family. This common activity gave the family an opportunity to experience some togetherness.

DISCUSSION

Our conclusions relate to: (a) the structure and process of the interventions; (b) the content of the interventions and the techniques which were implemented; and (c) the context of the interventions, that is, the Social Services Departments.

(a) The Structure and Process of the Interventions

Interventions with multiproblem, or FED, families should be multilevel and ought to include under case management such items as financial assistance, advocating, mediating, and family therapy. We are not convinced that concentrating only on family therapy, even with a variety of approaches and techniques, suffices when intervening with multiproblem families. This population needs help in communicating and connecting with different institutions in the community. Therefore, advocating and mediating are an integral part of the intervention process. Ignoring this aspect of intervention does not allow the family to concentrate on the emotional and functional issues that arise during family therapy.

It is important that the interventions be implemented by a therapeutic team and not by one social worker. Working as a team allows a definition and sharing of roles that are required when intervening with FED families. The team presents the family with a model of communication. However, the most important thing is that the team prevents the development of a coalition of despair between the social worker and the family (Shamai, 1989).

The focus and the target of the interventions are the functioning of individual members in the family. Therefore, it is important that all members of the family take part in the meetings and not only the wives/mothers (as is usually the case in Social Services Departments). Focusing on the family functioning, rather than on personality changes, seems to be more effective and leads to a higher probability of success in working with FED families.

We recommend structured and short-term interventions because multiproblem families have difficulties in organizing themselves for long, open-ended, unstructured therapy without a clear goal. The intervention design should be structured and short-term, with approximately ten meetings. After the initial period of intensive interventions, it is important to let the family internalize the change, practice and maintain it. After a few months, it is possible to begin another series of intensive structured short-term interventions.

We suggest meeting the family in their own home in order to remove from them the burden of organizing all the family members to arrive on time at the Social Services Department. We assume that holding sessions at home reduces cancellations of meetings and may even be critical in allowing the interventions to take place.

(b) The Content of the Interventions and the Techniques Used

We found that special attention must be paid to the balance of power between the spouses. Due to social stereotypes, many of the women had been perceived by the social workers as weak while their husbands had been perceived as strong. During the project, the impression of the family therapists about the power balance between the spouses was different from that of the social workers. We found that the majority of the women were stronger than their husbands in their level of functioning as well as in their verbal ability. The role and status of the women in their family life was prominent and secure. This significant role of the women allowed their husbands very limited access to influence the family. The limited and insignificant role of the husbands thus became another reinforcement for the escape from responsibility that characterized many of the men in the FED families.

It is important to use the therapeutic intervention as a device for balancing power between the spouses so that both the husbands and the wives can experience and express power in ways conducive to improving the functioning of the family. It is possible that the women, who used to be central to the family's relationship with the social workers, will express their resistance to sharing power in the family.

The issue of parenting is relevant to the majority of the families and can be a good way to join and create a therapeutic contract with the family. Relating to parental issues allows the staff to work with the parents as a team and to circumvent the fear of many families about discussing marital issues. We found that it was important to have the children participate in the therapeutic sessions. For many children, the meetings were good models for discussion and decision-making. In many families, the therapeutic sessions were the only times when the children received direct attention from their parents. Since many of the FED families had large numbers of children, we advised that they be divided into groups by their ages and be invited accordingly to meetings. By doing so, we increased the individuation of each child and enhanced the opportunity to focus on specific interaction patterns among family members.

Sometimes it may be necessary to remove a child from home. It is important that such a step be perceived as nonpunitive both by the parents and the child. It is the duty of the social worker to support the connection between the parents and the foster family or the institution where their child is placed, so that the child's feeling of rejection and the parents' feelings of failure will be lessened. Placing a child in a foster home or an institution does not mean creating a distance between the child and his or her family, nor need it necessarily remove responsibility from the parents.

Central issues in intervening with FED families are: creating boundaries that facilitate the organization of the family; reducing the chaotic situation; promoting communication that includes negotiation about roles and rules in the family, and if at all possible, about emotional issues as well.

Regarding the different techniques that have been utilized, it is important to indicate that in contrast with the populations researched in the literature of the 1960s, the families in our project were capable of using cognitive techniques and procedures. In addition, it is possible to integrate such techniques into the therapeutic interventions in conjunction with behavioral and creative techniques.

(c) The Context of the Interventions– The Social Services Departments

The Social Services Department is the "family" of the social worker. Without this supporting resource, it is possible that many of the social workers would feel disappointment and despair in working with FED families. The Social Services Department should create a supporting system for the social workers. This can be achieved by allowing intervention of a team, such as two workers with each family, by showing interest in their work, and by giving ongoing supervision.

All these can prevent the despair of social workers and increase their skills in coping with the challenge of working with FED families.

Finally, we would like to stress the fact that this model is costly in the short-term, since it requires some major policy changes to meet the financial and manpower demands:

   a. Training FED workers to be qualified in family therapy techniques and multi-professional teamwork.
   b. Reorganizing intervention strategies vis-à-vis the selection of FED cases and the assignment of at least two workers per family.
   c. Providing intensive supervision and consultation to the FED workers.
   d. Allowing additional financial assistance to meet specific needs according to the treatment goals.

However, it is our conviction that changes in the functioning of the family and in the motivation of the social workers would make this approach feasible in the long run.

Furthermore, we would like to reemphasize that top priority should be given to FED in order to break the vicious circle of poverty. Some of the differences found between the multiproblem families of past decades and the families in extreme distress being seen today are that the latter involve younger parents and more children per family (Sharlin, Katz, and Lavee, 1991). This situation, combined with the fact that the number of FED is rapidly increasing, underscores the need for additional resources to be allocated to this pressing problem.

CONCLUSION

This project supports different reports from the literature that it is possible to intervene in multiproblem families with positive results. We have developed several means of intervention with families in extreme distress. The families' and staff members' summaries of these interventions indicate that they were effective in creating changes in family functioning in several areas. However, in planning interventions with this population, it is important to provide a support system for the social workers and allow for constant reevaluation of the situation.

Our experience shows that investing the right resources was worthwhile. It is important to further test our conclusions and investigate whether their ramifications can be extended to similar interventions with other multiproblem families. We will continue to work on improving other modes of intervention while maintaining the hope that they will be used by social workers and other professionals who meet with such FED families.

REFERENCES

Aponte, H. (1974). Organizing treatment around the family's problems and their structural bases. *Psychiatric Quarterly, 48*, 209-222.

Aponte, H. (1976a). The family-school interview: An eco-structural approach. *Family Process, 15*, 303-311.

Aponte, H. (1976b). Underorganization in the poor family. In P. J. Guerin (Ed.) *Family therapy: Theory and practice.* New York: Gardner Press.

Aponte, H. (1986). If I don't get simple, I cry. *Family Process, 25*, 531-548.

Argles, P. & Machenzie, M. (1970). Crisis intervention with a multi-problem family: A case-study. *Journal of Child Psychology & Psychiatry & Applied Disciplines, 11*, 187-195.

Aronson, H. & Overall, B. (1966). Treatment expectations of patients in two social classes. *Social Work, 11*, 35-41.

Bandler, R. & Grinder, J. (1979). *Frogs into princess: Neuro linguistic programming.* Moab, UT: Real People Press.

Baum, O. E., Felzer, S. B., D'zmura, T. L. & Shumaker, E. (1966). Psychotherapy dropout and low socioeconomic patients. *American Journal of Orthopsychiatry, 36,* 629-635.

Beck, D. F. (1976). Research findings on the outcomes of marital counseling. In D. H. L. Olson (ed.) *Treating Relationships.* Lake Mills, IA: Graphic.

Bergin, A. E. & Lambert, M. J. (1978). The evaluation of therapeutic outcomes. In S. L. Garfield and A. E. Bergin (Eds.) *Handbook of psychotherapy and behavior change: An empirical analysis.* New York: Wiley & Sons.

Bernstein, V. J., Jeremy, R. J., Marcus, J. (1986). Mother-Infant interactions in multiproblem families: Finding those at risk. *Journal of American Academy of Child Psychiatry, 25,* 631-640.

Boscolo, L., Cecchin, G., Hoffman, L., Penn, P. (1987). *Milan systemic family therapy.* New York: Basic Books.

Coulshed, V. & Abdullak-Zedech, J. (1983). Case example of family therapy in social service department. *Social Work Today, 14,* 11-14.

Dax, E. C. & Hagger, R. (1977). Multiproblem families and their psychiatric significance. *Australian and New Zealand Journal of Psychiatry, 11,* 227-232.

Deutch, M. (1963). The disadvantaged child and the learning process. In A. H. Passow (Ed.) *Education in Depressed areas.* New York: Bureau of Publications, Teachers College, Columbia University.

Fischer, J. (1978). Effective casework practice: An eclectic approach. New York: McGraw-Hill.

Gans, H. G. (1963). Social and physical planning for the elimination of urban poverty. *Washington University Law Quarterly,* 2-18.

Garfield, S. L. (1978). Research of client variables in psychotherapy. In S. L. Garfield & A. E. Bergin (Eds.), *Handbook of psychotherapy and behavior change: An empirical analysis.* New York: Wiley & Sons.

Geismar, L. L. & La Sorte, M. A. (1964). Understanding the multiproblem family: A conceptual analysis and exploration in early identification. New York: Association Press.

Giordano, J. (1973). *Ethnicity and mental health.* New York: National Project on Ethnic America of the American Jewish Community.

Gould, R. E. (1967). Strangeclass: Or how I stopped worrying about the theory and began treating the blue-collar worker. *American Journal of Orthopsychiatry, 37,* 78-86.

Gurman, A. S. (1973). The effect and effectiveness of marital therapy: A review of outcome research. *Family Process, 12,* 145-170.

Hardy, F. C. & Macmahon, H. E. (1981). Adapting family therapy to the hispanic family. *Social Casework, 62,* 138-148.

Harrington, M. (1962). The other America: Poverty in the United States. New York: The Macmillan Co.

Heying, K. (1985). Family-based in home services for severely emotionally disturbed children. *Child Welfare, 5,* 519-527.

Hollingshead, A. B. & Redlich, F. C. (1958). *Social class and mental illness.* New York: Wiley.

Jenkins, H. (1983). A life-cycle framework in the treatment of underorganized families. *Journal of Family Therapy, 5*, 359-377.

Kaplan, M. L., Kurtz, R. M. & Clement, W. H. (1968). Psychiatric residents and lower-class patients: Conflict in training. *Community Mental Health Journal, 4*, 91-97.

Koegler, R. R. & Brill, N. Q. (1967). *Treatment of psychiatric outpatients.* New York: Appleton Century Crofts.

Lerner, B. (1972). *Therapy in the ghetto.* Baltimore: John Hopkins University Press.

Lewis, O. (1959). *Five families.* New York: Basic Books, Inc.

Lewis, O. (1961). *The children of Sanchez.* New York: Random House.

Lorion, R. P. (1973). Socioeconomic status and traditional treatment approaches reconsidered. *Psychological Bulletin, 79*, 263-270.

Lorion, R. P. (1978). Research on psychotherapy and behavior change with the disadvantaged: Past, present and future directions. In S. L. Garfield & A. E. Bergin (Eds.) *Handbook of psychotherapy and behavior change: An empirical analysis.* New York: Wiley & Sons.

Malone, C. A. (1963). Some observation of children of disorganized families and problem of acting out. *Journal of Child Psychiatry, 2*, 22-49.

Mannino, F. V. & Shore, M. F. (1972). Ecological oriented family intervention. *Family Process, 11*, 499-505.

Miller, S. M. (1964). The American lower class: A typological approach. In F. Reissman, J. Cohen & A. Pearl (Eds.) *Mental health of the poor.* New York: Free Press.

Minuchin, S. (1974). *Families and family therapy.* Cambridge: Harvard University Press.

Minuchin, S., Montalvo, B., Guerney, B. G., Rosman, B. L. & Schumer, F. (1967). *Families of the slums: An exploration of their structure and treatment.* New York: Basic Books.

Minuchin, S. & Fishman, C. H. (1981). *Family therapy techniques.* Cambridge, MA: Harvard University Press.

Parloff, M. B., Waskow, I. E., & Wolfe, B. E. (1978). Research on therapist variables in relation to process and outcome. In S. L Garfield, & A.E. Bergin (Eds.) *Handbook of psychotherapy and behavior change.* New York: Wiley & Sons.

Pavenstedt, E. (1965). A comparison of the child-rearing environment of upper-lower and very low-lower class families. *American Journal of Orthopsychiatry, 35*, 89-98.

Polansky, N. A., Borgman, R. D., DeSaix, C., & Smith, B. I. (1970). Two modes of maternal immaturity and their consequences. *Child Welfare, 49*, 312-323.

Polansky, N. A., Borgman, R. D., DeSaix, C., & Sharlin, S. (1971). Verbal accessibility in the treatment of child neglect. *Child Welfare, 50*, 349-356.

Polansky, N. A., Borgman, R. D. & DeSaix, C. (1972b). *Roots of futility.* San-Francisco: Jossey-Bass.

Polansky, N. A., Chalmers, M. A., Buttenwieser, E., & Williams, D. P. (1981).

Damaged parents, an anatomy of child neglect. Chicago & London: The University of Chicago Press.

Polansky, N.A., DeSaix, C. & Sharlin, S. (1972a). *Child neglect: Understanding and reaching the parents.* New York: Child Welfare League of America.

Rabin, C., Rosenbaum, H. & Sens, M. (1982). Home-based marital therapy for multiproblem families. *Journal of Marital and Family Therapy, 8,* 451-461.

Reid, W. J. (1985). *Family problem solving.* New York: Columbia University Press.

Riessman, F., Cohen, J. & Pearl, A. (Eds.) (1964). *Mental health of the poor.* New York: Free Press.

Salig, A. L. (1976). The myth of the multiproblem family. *American Journal of Orthopsychiatry, 46,* 526-532.

Schlosberg, S. & Kagan, R. (1988). Practice strategies for engaging chronic multiproblem families. *Social Casework, 69,* 3-9.

Schneiderman, L. (1965). Social class, diagnosis and treatment. *American Journal of Orthopsychiatry, 35,* 99-105.

Seabury, B. A. (1976). The contract: Uses, abuses and limitations. *Social Work, 21,* 16-21.

Shamai, M. (1987). Structured contract vs. general agreement. Unpublished dissertation, S. S. S. A., Chicago: University of Chicago.

Shamai, M. (1989). *Who writes the stories of poor families.* Unpublished Presentation at the 1st. International Family Therapy Congress, Dublin, Ireland.

Shapiro, A. K. & Morris, L. A. (1978). Placebo effects in medical and psychological therapies. In S. L. Garfield and A. E. Bergin (Eds.) *Handbook of psychotherapy and behavior change: An empirical analysis.* New York: Wiley & Sons.

Sharlin, S., Katz, R. & Lavee, Y. (1991). *Family policy in Israel, Vol. 3.* The Center for Research and Study of the Family, University of Haifa.

Spiegel, J. P. (1959). Some cultural aspects of transference and countertransference. In J. H. Masserman (ed.) *Individual and familial dynamics.* New York: Grune & Stratton, Inc.

Starkie, K. (1984). Family therapy of domestic violence service delivery system. *Clinical Social Work Journal, 12,* 78-84.

Tomlinson, R. & Peters, P. (1981). An alternative to placing children: Intensive and extensive therapy with 'disengaged' families. *Child Welfare, 60,* 95-103.

Tomm, K. (1984). One perspective on the milan systemic approach: Part II. Description of Session Format, Interviewing Style and Interventions. *Journal of Marital and Family Therapy, 10,* 253-271.

Weitzman, J. (1985). Engaging the severely dysfunctional family in treatment. *Family Process, 24,* 373-385.

Wells, S. J. (1981). A model of therapy with abusive and neglectful families. *Social Work, 26,* 113-118.

Yamamoto, J. & Goin, M. K. (1966). Social class factors relevant for psychiatric treatment. *Journal of Nervous and Mental Disease, 142,* 332-339.

The Impact of New Medical Technologies in Human Reproduction on Children's Personal Safety and Well-Being in the Family

Ruth Landau

SUMMARY. By nature and law, parents are expected to be the guardians and protectors of their children. Yet, evidence is available that the majority of children at risk are victimized by those who should protect them: their closest family.

Parenthood is a desired and valued task by individuals and society, and the new medical technologies in human reproduction assist individuals and couples to realize their wish for parenthood. Regretfully, they also create new and unprecedented forms of risk to childrens' personal safety and well-being in their family. The purpose of this paper is to show how children's personal safety and well-being in the family are affected by the circumstances under which their conception has occurred, and that use of modern technologies in the process of human reproduction may lead to child maltreatment, abuse, neglect or abandonment. Thus, societal intervention may be necessary in order to obviate the scope of these social phenomena.

INTRODUCTION

Parental status and roles are valued and desired nowadays by almost every woman and man. However, individuals and couples

Ruth Landau is Head of the Israeli Association of Planned Parenthood.

[Haworth co-indexing entry note]: "The Impact of New Medical Technologies in Human Reproduction on Children's Personal Safety and Well-Being in the Family." Landau, Ruth. Co-published simultaneously in *Marriage & Family Review* (The Haworth Press, Inc.) Vol. 21, No. 1/2, 1995, pp. 123-135; and: *Exemplary Social Intervention Programs for Members and Their Families* (ed: David Guttmann, and Marvin B. Sussman), The Haworth Press, Inc., 1995, pp. 123-135. Multiple copies of this article/chapter may be purchased from The Haworth Document Delivery Center [1-800-3-HAWORTH; 9:00 a.m. - 5:00 p.m. (EST)].

do not share the same destiny in this regard: by nature, some of the couples face pregnancy and birth more frequently than intended, while others need to cope with difficulties in order to achieve parenthood. This inequality is the reason why humankind from its beginning has intervened in human reproduction.

Behind all the new technologies in human reproduction there are good intentions: to help individuals and couples to exercise their will regarding reproduction and parenthood. Nevertheless, the implications of these medical advances which can limit the number of pregnancies and births, to overcome many of the difficulties stemming from infertility, and save lives by use of tissue or organ transplants, are not necessarily congruent with the children's best interest.

In some societies, cultures and groups, if family planning methods are not practised, children may be exposed to situations in which their basic needs are unmet. In contrast where birth control is carefully used, or the pregnancy and birth are achieved by means of "assisted conception" technologies, there may be danger for children.

Such children are intended, wanted, and probably rare. Thus, their arrival may be marked by too many expectations.

THE DESIRE FOR THE "PERFECT" CHILD

The risk to the personal safety and well-being of children in the family does not stem only from the lack of family planning. On the other end of the planning continuum are those families where children are planned and wanted. The fact that they are planned, and relatively rare, does not prevent them from being exposed to risks to their well-being. Good intentions expose them to a longer series of different interventions, medical and educational, some of them traumatic.

The new discoveries in the field of human reproduction allow the prevention, treatment and correction not only of children's but also fetuses' physical handicaps, and conception and parenthood occurs in cases that only 15 years ago would be unthinkable. Because they are wanted and carefully planned, "children gradually cease to be accepted as they are, with their specific physical and mental shortcomings" (Beck-Gernsheim, 1990, p. 453). As the author writes, the aim now is to correct every deficiency (no more stuttering, bed-wetting), and to develop every possible disposition (piano lessons, tennis and ski courses, linguistic holidays), with the abundant help of books, periodicals and professional guidance experts. Consequently, in a very deterministic way, parents are believed to be able to raise a "perfect" child. In other words, it is the expectation of the parents themselves and society to produce a perfect product.

In view of the above, Beck-Gernsheim (1990) raises the following questions: What will be the consequences for parenthood and, in particular, for the "norm of responsible parenthood?" Will the responsible parents of the future still be prepared to accept the fact that their children may have a handicap? Should they make sure that no impairment exists? Parents who accept the requirement to produce a perfect child need to make use of all the instruments of prenatal diagnosis. The greater the possibility for early detection of defects in the fetus, the more decisions to terminate the pregnancy should be expected. Any other choice would mean acceptance that the child would from the outset have less favourable opportunities in life. Beck-Gernsheim raises the issue whether parent's duty in the future will include answering the question as to whether "hereditary material" meets societal requirements.

However, the prenatal diagnosis required nowadays reflects the social control exercised on parents to comply. The aim is to give birth and raise a child without impairments. Consequently, induced abortions based on medical reasons are more frequent even in cases where only minor damage is anticipated. Similarly, social control is exercised as parents are required to follow a series of interventions to assure a newborn's health. There is more knowledge of children than ever before, according to Sommerville (1990), but it is largely confined to professionals. Socially and geographically mobile couples are separated from the experience and advice of their own parents and even where they are not, scientific ways of child care are deemed superior to the folk knowledge passed between generations (Hart, 1987). As Sommerville (1990) contends, "the very fact that there are experts may be intimidating; we hate to think that there must be one best way to handle any situation as parents and that we don't know what it is. So as we get more and more advice we seem less and less sure of what we ought to do for our children" (p. 5). Therefore, even after getting the advice it may not be used; or due to lack of confidence it may be unsought or even consciously avoided. In these cases parents are perceived as failures in their parental role (Dinai and Lahav, 1989). Thus, the impact of the new technology helps to set new standards for human perfection or human defects, where as the desire to have a healthy baby is now giving way to pressure to have a perfect child (Beck-Gernsheim, 1990).

So, if the parents fail to fulfill their duties in either phase of parenthood, before or after birth, they may face the reality of a less than perfect child. Such a child may, obviously, also be the consequence of a failure of the new technological procedures. However, if the expectations for a perfect child are so profound, what kind of reaction may be expected of parents whose child does not fit this new form? If they did follow all the directions, they may feel deceived, deprived and frustrated. Thus, if the product of the planned pregnancy is either impaired or in any other form incompatible with the most innate wishes of the parents, should it come as a surprise that abuse, neglect or abandonment may follow? In Israel, in a study conducted during a period of six years in three hospitals, annually about 30 imperfect infants are reported to be abandoned by their parents in these hospitals (Weiss, 1991). Due to gender planning–another achievement of the modern medical advances–7999 of 8000 induced abortions performed after prenatal sex determination were of female fetuses, according to a study in India (Sachar et al., 1990).

AIDS TO FERTILITY

The prevalence of infertility among couples in the developed countries is between 10 to 15 percent (WHO, 1989), and is increasing. The societal trend of delayed marriage and childbirth is associated with the increasing incidence of infertility. Increasing age in women is associated with a higher prevalence of pelvic disease and longer use of birth control methods with possible subsequent hormonal disturbances. As men get older, according to the WHO (1989) publication, they increasingly risk exposure to harmful environmental agents and drugs and the likelihood increases of contracting diseases that can also reduce fertility. Nearly one-quarter of all men are affected due to exposure to chemicals, radioactive materials, etc., (Edwards, 1991). Various factors can affect health as couples age and reduce their fertility. However, it is not only the number of infertile couples which is increasing but also the number of these couples seeking help, particularly due to the availability of the new medical technologies in the field (WHO, 1989).

Couples' needs to reproduce gave legitimacy to almost all means available to achieve pregnancy, birth and child. Artificial insemination, in vitro fertilization and surrogate parenthood, all characterized by lack of clarity as to the parents' identity when donor is involved, introduce another line of possible breach of parental responsibility and child protection. Lack of clarity in this regard may complicate the bond between parent and child, and eventually also weaken the incest taboo.

As Stanworth (1987) indicates, to those who see sex, marriage and parenthood as a dissoluble triad, the new medical technologies in human reproduction offer a dangerous precedent. They separate parenthood from the "sexual act," and do not ensure that parenthood will be confined to marriage. Furthermore, these technologies create a demand for children by single women, both heterosexual and lesbian (Edwards, 1991). Similar behavior on the part of men should be expected in the near future if surrogate motherhood becomes more available.

Daniels (1989) and Edwards (1991) raise questions regarding the origins, identity, rights and the quality of relationships in the family of children conceived by use of these new technologies. In a rather controversial way, the new medical technologies, while thriving on the cultural pressures towards having a child "of our own," also place the whole notion of parenthood in jeopardy (Stanworth, 1987). This is occurring at a time when embryologists and obstetricians are needed to bring about insemination and conception. Genetic parenthood no longer seems a "natural" process.

Thus, according to Stanworth, the new reproductive technologies carry the threat (or the promise) of delegitimation of the genetic parenthood and even of fracturing commonsense understanding of what is "the biological."

While the advances in medical technologies in the area of human reproduction are fast, Sweden is the first country where the issue of children's personal safety and well-being from this perspective has been legally addressed. The following measures in this respect were legally defined in Sweden in 1985 (Bygdeman, 1989):

1. Insemination by donor or husband as a medical treatment can be used only if the mother is married or cohabitating with a man. Moreover, written consent is required from the husband or the cohabiting man. Single women are excluded from this treatment. The reason for this is that it is considered important for the child's development to grow up in a complete family.
2. In order to give children born following insemination by donor the best possible conditions, the child's rights to know the donor's identity were provided. Children born after insemination by donor have to be informed so that they can find out the donor's name.
3. The treatment could be given only in general hospitals where not only the doctor but also a representative of the social welfare and a psychologist investigate whether the requested treatment is a suitable one. This procedure provides these children the same legal status as biological and adopted children have.

   It should be indicated that the medical experts in Sweden agreed with these measures but were overruled. It should be noted that the number of artificial inseminations by donors have decreased. Believing that to have children can never be an unconditional human right, and that the best interests of children must be secured, Sweden also has, since 1 January 1989, a law covering in vitro fertilization. Conditions are similar as for insemination with the exception that the ovum be the woman's own and be fertilized with sperm from her husband or cohabiting partner (Sverne, 1990).

According to the less strict United Kingdom Human Fertilization and Embryology Act 1990–deemed by Kenneth Clark, then Secretary of State for Health, the most comprehensive measure of its kind in the world–in any decision relating to the provision of a regulated service, account must be taken of the welfare of any child who may be born as a result of treatment, including the need of that child for a father (Snowden, 1992). The woman's husband or partner is regarded in all respects as the child's father, with one notable exception relating to inheritance, unless it is shown he did not consent to his partner's treatment.

The independent Human Fertilization and Embryology Authority, created to control and license centres offering "assisted conception" technologies, is required to keep a register which links any identifiable person to regulated infertility treatment. A person who is proved to have been born following infertility treatment has a right to receive certain limited information at the age of 18. However, unlike in Sweden, no donor identifying information can be made available. As Snowden (1992) notes, there are still those in the UK who believe that the rights of the child born following use of donated gametes have not been fully met due to the enforced anonymity of donors.

Sweden and UK, unlike other countries, have made serious attempts to regulate the issues posed by the new medical technologies in human reproduction. However, it is Sweden only that provides the child information about his or her origins and a legal status similar to that of biological children.

The general consensus that children's maltreatment is associated with elevated rates of insecure infant-mother attachments (Gelles and Conte, 1990). The new reproductive technologies, often characterized by lack of biological parenthood, may add more insecurity to the child-parent relationship. If, as Edwards (1991) believes, these innovations suggest that the family of the future may merely consist of one socialized adult and an offspring, children in the future may be deprived not only of their origins and identity, be exposed to maltreatment due to lack of secure child-parent attachment, but also experience growing up in single-parent families. Since children living in single-parent families are more likely to be poor than those in two-parent families (Aldous and Dumon, 1990), lack of clear biological (and legal) ties between child and parent may further erode the concepts of parental role and responsibility for the young.

Recently, artificial insemination using eggs from younger women and sperm of men enables the pregnancy of post-menopause women (Gorman, 1991). From a medical standpoint, there are two problems with late childbearing: health risks to the fetus and to the mother. After age 40, the risk of fetal abnormalities is substantial. The incidence of Down's Syndrome, for example, rises to 1 in 40 live births. The mother meanwhile faces increased risk of diabetes, obesity, high blood pressure and other complications of pregnancy, all of which can harm the unborn child.

However, the ethical and social issues rising from these medical advances are not less serious. Is it too much to ask that a child be given the chance of having parents who, theoretically at least, are capable of raising a child, instead of having her or him to take care of them early in his life? Who is actually the mother of the child conceived this way? And who will take care and assume parental responsibility when the "child" conceived this way will be less than perfect?

Theoretically, there is no medical contraindication to pregnancy by means of in vitro insemination by donors. Does it mean that couples and individuals will be able to "order" measure-made children according to their wishes and preferences? Will they have the choice to contribute their eggs/sperms or to ask donors to do so? Will women have the choice between going through the experience of pregnancy and giving birth or having someone else to do this for them? Will this be done out of altruism or for financial benefits?

As noted by Edwards (1991), the Third World surrogate industry could emerge as a new stage in their colonization and exploitation by First World nations.

For whatever reasons these choices will be made, there will be less and less clarity as to the parents' identity and responsibility. And since even these new technologies are not perfect, the situation from the point of view of childrens' personal safety and well-being seems even more complicated when the planned "child" will not be as perfect as expected.

ORGAN TRANSPLANTATION

The new medical advances can nowadays save children's lives by organ transplants. However, as the number of children in need of organ transplants increases, so does the demand for organs that can be used in transplantation. Cynthia Bell (1986) points out how in face of compelling medical need, prospective donors as well as prospective recipients are subject to strong pressures. Since a sibling who is a minor is often the most medically acceptable organ donor for a child needing an organ transplant, it cannot be assumed, according to Bell, that the best interests of the child donor are adequately protected by his parents.

The issue of parents' consent to tissue or organ donation by a child versus minor's right to consent is still not solved, but the new technologies in medicine pose even newer possibilities, and with them difficult questions. Is it ethical to plan the conception of a child with the clear purpose of having him to donate the necessary tissue or organ to his older siblings? The first baby conceived for this purpose has already occurred (Morrow, 1991). In the same line of argumentation, in extreme situations, children, who are unwanted, abandoned or unprotected, may be exposed to the risk of being abused or even killed for "spare parts" for those who are willing to pay.

REPRODUCTIVE TECHNOLOGIES AND THE MEDICAL PROFESSION

On the face of it, the medical profession does its utmost in order to assist individuals and couples to achieve their wish for parenthood. However, altruism is not the only value involved. As the demand for obstetric services in the developed countries has decreased, more and more physicians seem to be interested in infertility (WHO, 1989).

For obstetricians and gynecologists, the new reproductive technologies may mean high-status area of research, increased funds they can command (Stanworth, 1987), job-enrichment due to subspecialization such as foetal medicine and reproductive medicine (Pfeffer, 1987), fame and higher income.

Given these advantages it is not surprising that the present research orientation is for either more preventive or more curative medicine or both—more and more effective screening procedures, infertility clinics and gene therapies for imperfect organs or fetuses (Rose, 1987). Perhaps, as Rose contends, an alternative approach–

the ecological–is preferable. The ecological approach asks about the causes of the phenomena and demands less toxic environments, safe contraception, access to healthier lifestyles and for conditions that actively promote health.

This approach may be particularly useful in view of the limited extent to which questions about effectiveness, safety and social responsibility have been asked or answered regarding these new technologies (Oakley, 1987). The fact that these technologies are not evaluated before becoming part of routine medical practices reflects the lack of any systematic public control in this area. Oakley (1987) points out that the situation is even worsened by the commercial interests involved.

Thus, the new reproductive technologies are experiments without control, the medical and the social cost of which are still unknown. The wide use of X-rays as a means of monitoring pregnancy even twenty years after the publication of data showing an increased risk of childhood cancer following X-rays in utero, op. cit. Oakley (1987) indicates the primacy of the medical profession in the field on the one hand, and its neutrality, on the other. In view of the above, the question whether the assessment of risks and benefits of the use of these technologies can be left in the hands of the medical "experts" appears to be legitimate.

THE BEST INTEREST OF THE CHILD?

Many cases of children's maltreatment, abuse, neglect or abandonment can be traced back to as early as the stage of preconception. Use or nonuse of family planning methods, the reasons for this, the circumstances under which conception is achieved, the maturity for parenthood, and the quality of the relationship between the prospective parents of the child are factors that may affect children's personal safety and development in their families. The conscious and unconscious decisions made regarding parenthood are crucial for children's protection by those who are supposed to be their primary and first protectors: their own parents.

The issues raised in this article may have still not reached the stage of a social problem as defined by Herbert Blumer (1971): "social problems are fundamentally products of a process of collective definition instead of existing independently as a set of objective social arrangements with an intrinsic make up" (p. 298). But that the family has become a social problem is best illustrated by the Family Support Act of 1988 in the US. Due to separation between that which is public and that which is private, with the family considered the most private of social institutions, a separation between the family and government has been maintained throughout the American history (Rice, 1979). The Family Support Act of 1988 in the US reflects a major change in this respect. If the family, characterized by higher illegitimacy and divorce rates, "has begun to divest itself of the responsibility for the young" (Aldous and Dumon, 1990, p. 1143) when the young in question is a biological offspring, one wonders what will happen when no direct biological ties will connect child and parent.

CONCLUSION

Whereas major changes regarding family formations in the developed countries take place, the desire for parenthood is still prevalent. Individuals, young and older, heterosexual and homosexual, are willing to undergo stressful treatments with low rates of success in order to walk out the hospital with a "child of their own." The drive for a "biological" offspring, even by means of assisted conception technologies, coupled with the desire for a "perfect" child puts enormous pressure on those involved. The disappointments, when reality does not meet the expectations, may traumatically affect child-parent relationship.

Thus, the exponentially increasing medical advances in general, and the technologies in human reproduction in particular, create new and unprecedented forms of risk to children's personal safety and well-being in their family. According to the cultural lag theory, as formulated by Ogburn (1964), changes in nonmaterial culture, such as laws, beliefs and ideologies, tend to lag behind changes in material culture, such as technology. But since the issue discussed here may have an unforeseeable impact on society, perhaps as Beck-Gernsheim (1990) contends, the implementation of technologies should not be perceived as a natural law but as a social process which may be slowed down if that is felt appropriate.

Therefore, careful legislation, based on multidisciplinary intervention–excluding the primacy of the medical profession–may be necessary in order to protect the personal safety and well-being of children in their families.

Further research on the psychological and psychosocial aspects of the new medical technologies in human reproduction on various members of the family seems to be in need in general, and as a policy-making tool in particular.

Involvement of social scientists, social workers and family therapists–particularly specialists who encounter in their practices families and those whom society labels as "imperfect"–may provide a meaningful contribution in understanding the complicacy of the issues involved and the need to protect children even from their parents, prospective or present.

REFERENCES

Aldous, J. and Dumon, W. (1990). Family policy in the 1980s: Controversy and consensus. *Journal of Marriage and the Family*, 52, 1136-1151.

Beck-Gernsheim, E. (1990). The changing duties of parents: From education to bio-engineering? *International Social Science Journal*, 126: 451-463.

Bell, C. (1986). Children as organ donors. *Health and Social Work*.

Blumer, H. (1971). Social problems as collective behavior. *Social Problems*, 18.

Bygdeman, M. (1909). Swedish law concerning insemination. *IPPF Medical Bulletin*, 23(5): 3-4.

Daniels, K. R. (1989). Psychosocial factors for couples awaiting in vitro fertilization. *Social Work in Health Care*, 14(2): 81-90.

Dinai, A. and I. Lahav (1989). Mothers in a distressed neighborhood in view of the family health care clinic. *Society and Welfare*, 10(2): 133-147 (Hebrew).

Edwards, J. N. (1991). New conceptions: Biosocial innovations and the family. *Journal of Marriage and the Family*, 53: 349-360.

Gorman, C. (1991). When old is too old? *Time International, The Weekly Magazine*, 130(13), September 30.

Gelles, R. I. and Conte, J. R. (1990). Domestic violence and sexual abuse of children: A review of research on the eighties. *Journal of Marriage and the Family*, 52, 1045-1050.

Hart, N. (1987). The causes and consequences of the growth of technology in human reproduction. In L. Shamgar-Handelman and R. Palomba (Eds.) *Alternative patterns of family life in modern societies*, (pp. 351-374). Roma: Collana Monografie.

Morrow, L. (1991). When body can save another. *Time International, The Weekly Magazine*, 137(24), June 17.

Oakley, A. (1987). From walking wombs to test-tube babies. In Stanworth, M. (Ed.) *Reproductive technologies: Gender, motherhood and medicine.* Cambridge, UK: Polity Press.

Ogburn, W. F. (1964). *On culture and social change.* Chicago: University of Chicago Press.

Pfeffer, N. (1987). Artificial insemination, in-vitro fertilization and the stigma of infertility. In Stanworth, M. (Ed.) *Reproductive technologies: Gender, motherhood and medicine.* Cambridge, UK: Polity Press.

Rice, R. M. (1979). Exploring American family policy. *Marriage and Family Review* 2(3).

Rose, H. (1987). Victorian values in the test-tube: The politics of reproductive science and technology. In Stanworth, M. (Ed.) *Reproductive technologies: Gender, motherhood and medicine.* Cambridge, UK: Polity Press.

Sachar, R. K. et al. (1990). Sex selective fertility control–An outrage. *Journal of Family Welfare,* 36(2).

Snowden, R. (1992). The UK Human Fertilization and Embryology Act 1990. *IPPF Medical Bulletin,* 26(1): 3-4.

Sommerville, C. J. (1990). *The rise and fall of childhood.* New York: Vintage Books.

Stanworth, M. (1987). Reproductive technologies and the destruction of motherhood. In Stanworth, M. (Ed.) *Reproductive technologies: Gender, motherhood and medicine.* Cambridge, UK: Polity Press.

Sverne, T. (1990). Bio-technological developments and the law. *International Social Science Journal,* 126, 465-475.

Weiss, M. (1991). *Conditional love: Parental relations towards handicapped children.* Tel Aviv: Sifriat Poalim (Hebrew).

WHO (World Health Organization). (1989). *Guidelines on diagnosis and treatment of infertility.*

Stress Inoculation Training
for Stepcouples

Donald F. Fausel

SUMMARY. Stepfamilies do not have the corner on the market of having to cope with stress. However, there is ample evidence that the complexities of living in a stepfamily produce its own set of stressors that first families are not exposed to. Recent research identifies interpersonal stress as the major problem in all steprelationships (Martin & Martin, 1992; Stanton, 1986; Visher & Visher, 1982).

This paper examines the nature of stress in stepfamilies, describes a program for stepcouples designed to assist couples to deal with stress, Stress Inoculation Training (SIT) and evaluates the utility of SIT as experienced by fifty-one stepcouples. SIT was developed by Donald Meichenbaum and has been applied effectively to a number of diverse populations (Meichenbaum, 1985, pp. 24-25). The program reported in this paper was a collaborative effort between the School of Social Work at Arizona State University and East Valley Jewish Family and Children's service in Mesa, Arizona.

STEPFAMILIES AND STRESS

Stepfamilies

Data collected and analyzed by the National Center for Health Statistics suggest that stepfamilies continue to make up a significant

---

Donald F. Fausel is Professor in the School of Social Work, Arizona State University, Tempe, AZ.

[Haworth co-indexing entry note]: "Stress Inoculation Training for Stepcouples." Fausel, Donald F. Co-published simultaneously in *Marriage & Family Review* (The Haworth Press, Inc.) Vol. 21, No. 1/2, 1995, pp. 137-155; and: *Exemplary Social Intervention Programs for Members and Their Families* (ed: David Guttmann, and Marvin B. Sussman) The Haworth Press, Inc., 1995, pp. 137-155. Multiple copies of this article/chapter may be purchased from The Haworth Document Delivery Center [1-800-3-HA-WORTH; 9:00 a.m. - 5:00 p.m. (EST)].

proportion of the total number of marriages. According to the publications from the Center, of the two million couples married each year in the 1980s, more than 40% of these marriages were remarriages for one or both spouses (National Center for Health Statistics, 1991). In 1988, almost 1.5 million divorced women and men remarried in the United States (Wilson & Foley, 1992).

There are a number of sources of stress in stepfamilies that are not found in other families. One of the most severe is the fact that the stepfamily is born out of the loss of the first family and the single-parent family. For the stepfamily to be successful, it is necessary for its members to mourn the loss of the first and single-parent family (Sager et al., 1983). It is also necessary that family members learn to negotiate new relationships that are not found in first marriages, such as between stepparent and stepchildren; to renegotiate parenting arrangements with a birth parent, who perhaps has not dealt with his/her anger around the divorce and has a vested interest in seeing that his/her spouse's new relationship fails. When these tasks are not accomplished, the chances of the stepfamily thriving and surviving is minimal. Despite the fact that 50% of first marriages dissolve without the additional stressors that first families experience (Goldenberg & Goldenberg, 1990), it is not surprising that remarried families are more likely to divorce than first families (Booth, & Edwards, 1992).

Add to the interpersonal issues mentioned above, ambiguities of roles, rules, boundaries, power issues, value differences and poor communications carried over from the first marriage, and stress entering the system is predictable (Fausel, 1981). Given these stressors, and a lack of preparation and institutionalization of the role of the stepperson (Cherlin, 1978), the fact that sixty percent of second marriages fail is a disturbing reality (*Behavior Today*, 1988). Perhaps Furstenberg and Spanier (1984), are correct in their hypothesis that second marriages are more likely to fail, not because of the Cherlin hypothesis of poorly defined roles, but because people who have been divorced once may be less committed to remaining in an unhappy marriage than those in a first marriage. Nevertheless, a sixty percent failure rate for second marriages is high and alarming (National Center for Health Statistics, 1991).

Although "stepfamily" has been used synonymously with "remarried," "blended," "reconstituted," and at least fourteen other names to describe this type of family structure (Wald, 1981), each synonym creates its own problems. For example, since the adults may not be married, only cohabiting, not all stepfamilies are "remarried" families. Also, terms such as blended or reconstituted do not define relationships. It would be ludicrous for a stepparent to introduce a child as "my blended child," or "my reconstituted child." So despite the negative connotation that "step" has from such sources as Cinderella and Snow White, for the purposes of this paper we will use the term stepfamily, and define it as: one in which children live some, most, or all of the time with two married or cohabiting (cohabiting added) adults, one of whom is not the biological parent (Stanton, 1986).

Stress

Stress has become the fashionable "disease" of our time (Fausel, 1991). Although there are many definitions of stress, for our purposes it is defined as "a response of the organism to conditions that, either consciously or unconsciously, are experienced as noxious" (Donovan, 1987, p. 259). This definition, unlike those that focus exclusively on the environment, e.g., the stress of the work place, or the stress of raising stepchildren, is transactional. "It reflects the relationship between the person and the environment that is appraised by the person as taxing or exceeding his or her resources and as is endangering his or her well-being" (Meichenbaum, 1985, p. 3).

The list of approaches to treating and preventing stress is wide. Ethel Roskies (1987) has identified a number of approaches. She writes, ". . . massage, exercise, nutrition, progressive relaxation, meditation, biofeedback, social skills training, stress inoculation training are only a few of the better known ones" (Roskies, 1987, p. 27).

No one stress management approach is likely to be effective with all individuals. An approach that includes flexibility, a variety of techniques that depend on the needs of the population that is being addressed would seem to be the most effective (Wertkin, 1985). Since we do not have the luxury in this article to evaluate all the programs that address stress, we have chosen Stress Inoculation Training (Meichenbaum, 1985) to apply to stepcouples, because it does include a variety of techniques, is flexible and in comparative studies was found to be effective in increasing coping skills in a variety of settings, by helping people cope with different stress-related problems (Wertkin, 1985).

STRESS INOCULATION TRAINING PROCEDURES

Stress inoculation training is a generic term referring to a three-phase treatment program that combines elements of didactic teaching, Socratic discussion, cognitive restructuring, problem-solving, relaxation training, behavioral and imaginal rehearsal, self-monitoring, self-instruction, self-reinforcement, and environmental manipulation. The specific training techniques vary depending upon the client population the training focuses on (Meichenbaum, 1985).

Meichenbaum outlines seven goals for SIT:

1. Teach clients the transactional nature of stress and coping.
2. Train clients to self-monitor maladaptive thoughts, images, feelings, and behaviors in order to facilitate adaptive appraisals.
3. Train clients in problem-solving, that is problem-definition, consequences, anticipation, decision-making and feedback.
4. Model and rehearse direct-action, emotion-regulation and self-control coping skills.
5. Teach clients how to use maladaptive responses as cues to implement their coping repertoires.
6. Offer practice in in vitro imaginal and behavioral rehearsal and in vivo graded assignments that become increasingly demanding, and to nurture clients' confidence in and use of their coping repertoires.
7. Help clients acquire sufficient knowledge, self-understanding and coping skills to facilitate better ways of handling (un) expected stressful situations (p. 22).

Stress inoculation training consists of three phases:

1. The conceptualization phase where the primary focus is on establishing a collaborative relationship with individuals and on

helping them to better understand the nature of stress in
actional terms.
2. The skills acquisition and rehearsal phase. During this phase
clients are taught to develop and rehearse a variety of coping
skills.
3. The application and follow-through phase. Clients practice
coping skills both in vitro (imaginal and behavioral rehearsal
in training sessions) and in vivo (performing personal experiments in real life). Small manageable units of stress are induced in vitro and gradually in vivo.

Although application of SIT to stepfamily stress in this project
suggests a linear progression through various phases, in practice the
phases blend together. For example, although assessment and
education are the main focuses of the first phase, assessment is
ongoing throughout the other phases. There is a continual reassess-
ment and revision of goals. Participants receive frequent practice in
developing and using coping behaviors. The three phases are incor-
porated in the description that follows.

STRESS INOCULATION TRAINING
FOR STEPCOUPLES

The application of SIT to stepcouples was a collaborative effort
between East Valley Jewish Family and Children Services and the
School of Social Work at Arizona State University. The agency had
received a grant from East Valley Behavioral Health Association to
establish prevention programs. Given the agency's long standing
interest in working with stepfamilies, they contracted with the author of this article to develop and deliver a six-week program for
stepcouples. This article is reporting on the results of the delivery of
the program to eleven groups of stepcouples, over a period of eigh-
teen months. Fifty-one couples, 102 individuals, participated in the
eleven groups. The SIT program developed and used with those
stepcouples will be presented below.
As stated in the *Stress Inoculation Training Handbook for Stepcouples* (Fausel, 1992), the purpose of the program is to: "assist
stepcouples in handling the stress that is inherent in blending two

families with multiple relationships into one family; to assist in developing new skills and strategies designed to improve relationships, and create a solid family system" (p. 1). The program includes six units with six behavioral objectives. These units correspond to the different phases identified by Meichenbaum, listed previously. A booklet of twenty handouts developed for this program is provided to each participant. The handouts reinforce the educational aspect of the program. It is made very clear from the beginning, that although the program might be therapeutic it is not intended to be therapy, but education.

UNIT I. INTRODUCTION/GET ACQUAINTED/ FAMILY SYSTEM CONCEPTS/TASKS AND TASKS TO DEVELOP A STEPFAMILY

Objective: To create an atmosphere for adult learning. Identify the issues and tasks facing stepfamilies and the underlying concepts of the family as a system.

Activities: Participants and leaders introduce themselves and tell a little about their family composition and issues they would like to see covered during the six weeks. The leader explains the six-week program: gives a preview of what participants can expect in the individual units by going over the objectives in the outline participants have in their packets. He/she gives a rationale for choosing SIT, identifying stress as a major factor in stepfamilies. An additional opportunity is given for participants to add any issues that they would like to add to those identified by the leader. It is particularly important in the leader's introduction that he/she is able to share his/her experiences and expertise in the area of stepfamilies.

The leader then gives a mini-lecture on family systems, rules, roles, boundaries, etc., and on the tasks that are necessary to develop a solid stepfamily system. Discussion and interaction with other couples follow and a homework assignment is given. The assignment is to recall and discuss with spouse/partner the rules from their respective family of origin and how they have developed the rules in their present family.

UNIT II. STRESS INOCULATION TRAINING

Objective: Demonstrate the ability to apply the components of SIT to the in vitro and in vivo stepsituations.

Activities: After checking on the homework assignment, which usually generates discussion and interaction with other couples, the leader explains SIT and demonstrates in a mini-lecture, guided imagery, relaxation, and cognitive restructuring (self-talk). Handouts on relaxation and imagery techniques are gone over. An imagery exercise is done and the leader suggests that participants put the exercise on tape with appropriate background music, so they can practice the technique at home. After the exercise is completed, the group processes the experience.

Participants are asked to complete a "Stressful Stepfamily Events Hierarchy" form in which they rank current situations in their lives as stepparents that they find stressful. The events are given weight from 5 to 100. An item that is ranked relatively low might be, "Kids don't want to phone their father." An item that would rank high would be, "Former spouse is late with child support." Some twenty examples are given on a handout that participants can use as a guide in creating their own hierarchy of stressful events.

The leader then goes over a stress inoculation trackdown, which is basically a way of teaching cognitive restructuring, "self-talk," the A-B-Cs as designed by Ellis (1962) and refined by Beck (1976) and Meichenbaum (1985).

A. Activating event: "Former spouse is late picking up kids for the weekend."
B. Beliefs and self-talk about "A": "He's always late. It's awful and I can't stand it. He's a very bad person, he shouldn't have done this to me, he's made my life miserable."
C. Feelings and behaviors: Anger, fear, rage, lashing out at kids, frantic calls to ex-spouse.
D. Dispute your beliefs and self-talk. "He's usually on time. Life is more pleasant when he is on time. I would be satisfied if he were on time 80% of the time. I need to make it very clear to him/her what my expectations are."

After the process is gone over with a number of other examples from the hierarchy of events list, couples are given an opportunity to first practice as a couple, and then volunteers are selected to practice before the other participants.

The homework assignment is to practice either the deep relaxation or the imagery exercise during the week and construct a hierarchy of events list. During the next four weeks part of the homework assignment will be to continue the deep relaxation and to practice the ABCDs self-talk at least three times during the week.

UNIT III. PARENTING HIS/HERS AND OURS

Objective: Demonstrate ability to parent both step and birth children.

Activities: After discussing the successes and problems with the homework assignment participants view a video, "When Mom and Dad Break Up." The video is used as an aid to discussion. Participants discuss the issues of unresolved loss and grief that often play a major part in the behavior of children of divorce. Other issues that the video dramatizes are the loyalty issue that children experience in being part of two families; the feeling of responsibility for the breakup of the marriage and the insecurities that children experience as the adult caregivers in their lives struggle with their own issues.

In addition to struggling with the feelings and behaviors that are often precipitated by divorce or separation, stepparents struggle with many of the same parenting issues that birth parents experience. A mini-lecture is given on an Adlerian approach to parenting, as outlined in the Systematic Training for Effective Parenting (STEP) (Dinkmeyer & McKay, 1983). A handout, based on the STEP program, that describes the goals of misbehavior in children, as well as alternative responses on the part of parents, is discussed and processed. These goals, purposes and irrational beliefs underlying the behaviors apply equally to children in step or birth families. Couples are then asked to simulate situations that they might have experienced with their children and engage in problem-solving.

The homework assignment is to analyze their (step) child's behavior in terms of the goals of misbehavior and experiment with an alternative response suggested in the handout. For example, if their assessment is that their child is misbehaving to gain attention, they are to ignore the behavior and focus on giving attention for positive behavior.

UNIT IV. COMMUNICATION IN STEPFAMILIES

Objective: Demonstrate effective communication skills in the couple relationship and the parent-child relationship.

Activities: The leader asks for feedback on how the application of the alternative positive parenting techniques, discussed last week, worked. Following, what often is a lively discussion and suggestions from group members and leader how things might have been handled differently, if a particular approach didn't work, a mini-lecture is given on communications. Based on the assumption that poor communications is usually part of the problems families face and poor communications produce stress, the objective is to reduce stress by improving communications. A secondary objective is to clarify for couples that dealing with conflict is a necessary and legitimate part of intimacy and can be learned.

Handouts are distributed and discussed (Fausel, 1992) based on communication styles and basic communications skills (Satir, 1972), along with a couples communication exercise that Harville Hendrix calls "mirroring" (1988). Each couple is given an opportunity to practice the communication exercise in vivo, and receive feedback from the other participants. The purpose of this particular exercise is to help couples learn to listen to one another, bargain and negotiate for changes; resolve frustrations over important issues such as (step)parenting, sex, use of leisure time, etc.

Bargaining and negotiation are skills that couples often hadn't learned or applied in their first marriage (Hunter & Shuman, 1980). Often what they have learned, and carry over into second marriages is accommodation, and accommodation usually produces resentment and additional stress.

The homework assignment for the following week is to set aside time each day to practice the mirroring communication exercise. They are also given a copy of the "Stepparent Quiz" (Fausel, 1992), a series of twenty questions on issues related to steplife.

UNIT V. COUPLING

Objective: Demonstrate the ability to preserve and enhance the couple relationship despite the complexities of living in step.

Activities: Leader asks for feedback on the utility of the "mirroring" exercise. When couples have had difficulty implementing it during the week, this is discussed, and further in vivo practice is provided. The difficulties that others have had, is an opportunity for the whole group to learn from the couple that brings their problems to the group.

The leader then solicits from the group questions they might have had about particular questions on the "Stepfamily Quiz." Again, this usually provided a good springboard for discussion, since many of the questions in the quiz have no right or wrong answers, but are geared to stimulate discussion.

Since couples often lose sight of the importance of the couple relationship and become child-focused, particularly in stepfamilies (Larson & Allgood, 1987), participants are asked to evaluate their relationship. A handout, "Diagnose Your Relationship" (Luecke, 1981), which asks each individual to separately assess the couple relationship in four areas: (1) Cooperation, (2) Compatibility, (3) Intimacy, (4) Emotional Support, using a simple Likert-type scale. Couples are then asked to discuss how they scored each item and talk over the differences and similarities. Couples then share and receive feedback from the other participants.

The homework assignment is to: continue discussions of the Relationship Diagnosis with partner during the week; integrate the mirroring exercise in resolving any areas of difference; use the self-talk techniques when stress enters the system, and it becomes difficult not to fall back into old ways of dealing with conflict. The focus of the assignment is what each individual would like to see change in their relationship, rather than how they can be better (step)parents.

UNIT VI. FORMERLY SPOUSES, PARENTS FOREVER

Objective: Assist participants in working out visitation arrangements with former spouses in the best interest of the children.

Activities: Leader asks for self-report from couples on their ability to integrate the components of their homework assignment described above. Where there have been problems, the couple is given an opportunity to share with the group and get suggestions for handling situations differently. Feedback from group members has consistently been that this interaction with other couples is very helpful.

A handout (Fausel, 1992) on the principles of the binuclear family is distributed and discussed. The leader presents a mini-lecture based on *Mom's House, Dad's House* (Ricci, 1980), the typology of five parenting partnerships (Durst, Wedemeyer & Zurcher, 1985), and the binuclear family concept developed by (Ahrons, C., & Rodgers, 1987).

Using the Durst, Wedemeyer and Zurcher Typology (1985), couples share the type of parenting partnerships they have with their former spouse:

Type I. Mother and Nonparent Father.
Type II. Mother and Father as Friend.
Type III. Mother and Restricted Father, i.e.,
parental role of father is ambiguous.
Type IV. Time-Sharing Parents.
Type V. Co-parents, i.e., clear and flexible boundary
between the parental and former spousal
subsystems.

These distinctions and descriptions of post divorce families assist the couples in looking at tasks that need to be accomplished to become a binuclear family. Although the types as listed here, need further defining information suffice it to say that Type I through Type V reflect an increase of father-child contact and parental role performance across the families (Durst, Voigt, & Wedemeyer, 1985). Each situation presents its own individual issues, which participants are often struggling with and can relate to. For example, if the former spouses have a Type I relationship, the child might be struggling with abandonment issues, since his noncustodial birth parent has little or no involvement in parenting after divorce or separation. If the former spouses have a Type V partnership which allows for a continued cooperative parenting relationship the child might be experiencing stress over loyalty issues, or confusion over different rules in separate households. Discussion and group sharing are helpful in integrating previously learned skills.

Specific material from Isolina Ricci's book (1980) is discussed. One example would be her suggestion to keep the parenting partnership with former spouse on a business-like arrangement (we often do business with people we don't even like) by using memos to clarify changes in visitation arrangements. Participants often have suggestions that have worked for them and they share successes and failures with other participants.

The final twenty minutes of this last session are set aside to do the formal evaluation of the program; informally discuss what was helpful and what not; explain other services that the agency has for stepfamilies, such as groups for children, separate groups for stepmothers and stepfathers, stepcouple and family counseling; and plans to offer a "drop-in" group for stepcouples who have "graduated" from the SIT.

Finally the Index of Clinical Stress (Walmyr, 1992) which will be explained in the next section, is administered as a posttest.

METHODOLOGY

One hundred and two individuals, 51 couples, participated in eleven different six-week groups in which the six unit SIT program described above was taught. The rationale for using the SIT program was the assumption that since interpersonal stress is a major problem in all step-relationships (Stanton, 1986), stepcouples could profit from learning new skills for managing stress, with the long-term expectation that participants would have a higher probability of a satisfying stepfamily life. Had this been an experimental design, participants would have been randomly assigned to a six-week program using another approach. For example, a solution focused or group interaction approach might have been selected to compare with SIT.

The Index of Clinical Stress (ICS) (Walmyr, 1992) was used as a pre- and posttest. ICS is a twenty-five item self-administered scale that measures the magnitude of problems that clients have with personal stress (Abell, 1991). Although the scale can evaluate stress globally, it can be aimed at more specific situations, such as stress in stepfamilies, that may be making the client vulnerable to stress-related disorders or discomfort (Walmyr, 1992). In using ICS more specifically, participants are asked to complete the scale in terms of his/her stepfamily life.

ICS produces scores that range from 0 to 100. Although a published clinical cutting score is not available for ICS, our own clinical judgement suggests a cut-off score for clinical significance of 30, since ICS is so similar to the other Walmyr scales which use 30 as a cut-off. The scale has consistently achieved an Alpha coefficient of .90 or larger, and with respect to content, construct and factorial validity, it nearly always achieves validity coefficients of .60 or greater (Walmyr, 1992, p. 17).

In addition to the ICS pre- and posttest, a formal and informal evaluation, described under Evaluation, was done at the end of the six weeks. Also, the leader kept careful notes on the self-reports that couples made in reporting their homework assignments.

DEMOGAPHICS

Marital Status

Thirty-nine (76%) of the fifty-one couples were currently married at the time they participated in the program. Of the 12 (24%) who were not married, 9 (75%) were living together. All of the couples who were not married indicated that they were taking the SIT as a premarital class to prepare them for the complexities of living in a stepfamily. Two of those unmarried couples were married during the course of the program. One of those couples had been living together, and the other not. Another couple who had been living together decided to end their relationship. They reported that the SIT had helped them look at their situation more realistically and helped with the decision to separate. They reported that they were able to make a cleaner break because of the skills they had learned in the program.

Age of Couples

The average age of the participants, 33.4, was 3.4 years younger than the national figures. Men averaged almost three years older than the women. Women's average was 32.0 and men 34.8. This compares with an average age for men in second marriages of 38.6 and for women 35.0, as reported by the National Center for Health Statistics (1991).

Time Together

Thirty-seven (73%) had been coupled in their present relationship for less than a year, and none had been together for over two years. Nine (18%) had been together as a couple for less than six months. This supports statements that most of the couples made that they originally came to the class to prevent problems and find solutions before they got too stuck and things seemed insurmountable. Since most researchers suggest that it takes anywhere from two to five years for a stepfamily to become a family and work through some of the complexities of forming a new family, the fact that these families have had so little time together might contribute to higher stress scores (Visher & Visher, 1978).

Interval to Remarriage

Fourteen (28%) of the women had less than nine months between their last marriage (or cohabitation/relationship) and their present marriage (or cohabitation/relationship), compared to thirty-seven (63%) of the men. The interval to remarriage for both men and women is far less than the 3.6 years for men and the 3.9 years reported for women reported by Wilson and Clarke, (1992). It could also be hypothesized that the shorter time between marriages could contribute to stress.

Number of Children

There was a total of 154 birth children between the participants. Women had 93 birth children from prior relationships, and men 59, and two children were from present relationships. Since negotiations over stepchildren account for a portion of the stress and decline in marital quality (Booth & Edwards, 1992) it could be hypothesized that couples with more complex stepchild(ren) configurations would experience more stress.

Custody Arrangements

It is apparent that custody distribution with these couples favored the birth mothers. Forty-three (84%) of the women were birth parents. Of those forty-three mothers, 42 (98%) had primary custody. Thirty-six (71%) of the men were birth parents. Of those thirty-six fathers, 11 (31%) had primary custody. Two of the fifty-one couples had children, one each, of their own. Obviously, a much higher percentage of men (29%) versus women (16%) came into the step or quasi-step relationship with no children. Men who have not had children of their own, and enter a family as a stepfather, tend to be overly involved in setting and enforcing rules with their new stepchildren than those who have had their own children (Visher & Visher, 1978). It also suggests a concern expressed by Marsiglio (1992), that stepfathers who have extremely high expectations for their children to follow rules and be obedient may have a more stressful time stepparenting than stepfathers with more moderate expectations.

Child Support

Twenty-five (60%) of the 42 women with primary custody of their children were receiving child support, compared to none of the eleven men. Twenty-two (88%) of the twenty-five men who did not have custody claimed they were paying child support to former partners, while the one woman who did not have primary custody was not paying child support. Based on these reports, the figures for both women receiving child support from former spouses and men providing support to their children from former relationships are high. This might be accounted for by the short period of time the spouses have been separated. The compliance with court ordered child support seems to decrease over time (Cassetty, 1984).

EVALUATION

Four methods of evaluation were used to assess whether the program met its goals and objectives: a formal evaluation form completed by participants; informal feedback from participants; observation of the leader and analysis of the pre- and post-ICS scores.

Written Evaluation

A written evaluation was given to participants at the end of each six-week program. Fifty-eight (57%) completed the form, which used a Likert-type scale to evaluate the program. The form included seven scaled questions and three open-ended questions. On a scale of 1-5, five being high, the overall evaluation of the program was 4.3. All participants agreed that the program was helpful. The rating for usefulness of the interaction with other couples was 4.5; the leader's helpfulness, 4.4; helpfulness of handouts and meeting goals and objectives, both were 4.0; and whether they would recommend the program to other stepparents, 4.5.

Informal Feedback

The feedback after each homework assignment was particularly helpful to the leader in assessing whether the skills taught in class were working. The in vivo practice in class offered another opportunity to judge whether or not what was being "taught was caught." Since the author taught all of the classes, he could give instant feedback on material that had not been integrated the first time.

Typical statements made by participants at the end of the six weeks, were, "I wish the six weeks were not up." "I wish there was a stepparenting 102 course." "I don't feel like the lone ranger anymore." "I feel much more confident in being a stepparent."

Index of Clinical Stress

Ninety-nine of the 102 individuals that participated completed the ICS as a pretest. Sixty-four (65%) were above the clinical cutting score of 30. Assuming accurate and candid responses, it can be presumed that only 35 (35%) of participants were free of clinically significant stress in their stepfamily relationships. This supports the assumption of this research, that stepcouples participating in this program would test high on the stress scale. Clearly, given the nature of this study and the self-selected sample, no broader conclusions can be drawn, but it does support the previously mentioned research that identified stress as being a, if not the, major issue in stepfamilies (Martin & Martin, 1992; Visher & Visher, 1982; Stanton, 1986).

Comparing the 74 who completed the ICS both before and after the six-week classes, forty-six (62%) scored lower on the posttest. Twelve (16%) of the forty-six participants whose ICS scores were lower in the posttest reduced their scores below the cutting score of 30. Although there are obviously a number of intervening variables that might account for cumulative reduction in scores, it would appear that the program was effective in reducing stress for a significant number of participants.

CONCLUSIONS

The purpose of this project was to deliver a program to stepcouples based on the assumption that they experience high stress and could learn new coping skills by participating in SIT, thus reducing their stress. The descriptive data suggest that the assumptions were correct. Sixty-five percent of the participants scored above the cut-off score of clinician significance on the pretest, and of the seventy-four who completed the posttest, sixty-two percent had reduced their stress scores.

We do not presume to imply a causal relationship between the participation in the SIT program and the reduction in ICS scores, but only suggest that further research, using a more experimental design, is indicated. Had an experimental group been used to compare the SIT program, (for example, this author is currently using a solution-focused approach and a pure discussion, no formal didactic content format) pre- and posttest scores would be compared for both comparison and experimental groups on the dependent measure of ICS by computing t-tests.

Without the comparison groups, it did not seem economical to do more analysis on the variables described earlier; age, number of children, etc., as they may or may not effect the presence or reduction of stress. Another flaw in the design of the project was that information was not collected on several major variables, specifically, educational and socioeconomic levels of participants. These variables can prove to be important and need to be considered in an experimental design (Wilson & Clarke, 1992).

The value of this project was more in designing the program to adapt SIT to the step-population and getting some preliminary feedback from the participants, so that this adaptation could be used by other practitioners. It would appear from the feedback from the participants, that the program, with its six units and twenty-handout manual was helpful to the majority of the participants.

REFERENCES

Abell, J. N. (1991). The index of clinical stress: A brief measure of subjective stress for practice and research. *Social Work Research & Abstracts*, 27, 2, 12-15.

Ahrons, C. & R. Rodgers (1987). *Divorced families: A multidisciplinary developmental view*. NY: Norton.

Beck, A. T. (1976). *Cognitive therapy and emotional disorders*. NY: International Universities.

Behavior Today, (1988). Changing family structures, 19, 1.

Booth, A., & Edwards, J. N. (1992). Starting over: Why remarriages are more unstable. *Journal of Family Issues*, 13, 179-194.

Cassetty, J. (1984). Child support: Emerging issues for practice. *Social Casework*, February.

Cherlin, A. (1978). Remarriage as an incomplete institution. *American Journal of Sociology*, 86, 634-650.

Christensen, O. & T. Scharmanski (Eds.) (1983). *Adlerian family counseling: A manual for counselors, educators, and psychotherapists*, Minneapolis, MN: Educational Media Corp.

Dinkmeyer, D. & G. McKay (1983). *Systematic training for effective parenting*. Circle Pines, MN: American Guidance Service.

Donovan, R. (1987). Stress in the workplace: A framework for research and practice. *Social Casework*, 68, 259-266.

Durst, P., Voigt, N., & Zurcher, L. (1985). Parenting partnership after divorce: Implication for practice. *Social Work*, Sept.-Oct. 1985.

Ellis, A. (1962). *Reason and emotion in psychotherapy*. NY: Lyle Stuart.

Fausel, D. F. (1981). Social work practice with reconstituted families, unpublished paper, *Seventh NASW Conference*, Philadelphia, PA.

Fausel, D. F. (1991). Supervision. In Allison Lewis et al., *Collaboration II: The supervisor*. Office of Human Development services, Award No. 09CW0954.

Fausel, D. F. (1992). *Stress inoculation training handbook for stepfamilies*, unpublished material, available through Arizona State University, School of Social Work.

Furstenberg, F. F., & G. Spanier. (1984). The risk of dissolution in remarriage: An examination of Cherlin's Hypothesis of incomplete institutionalization. *Family Relations*, 33, 433-441.

Goldenberg, H., & I. Goldenberg (1990). *Counseling today's families*. Pacific Grove, CA: Brooks/Cole.

Hendrix, H. (1990). *Getting the love you want: A guide for couples*. NY: Harper & Row.

Hunter, J. E., & Schuman, N. (1980). Chronic reconstitution as a family lifestyle. *Social Work*, July, 446-451.

Larson, J. H., & Allgood, S. (1987). A comparison of intimacy in first-married and remarried couples. *Journal of Family Issues*, 8, 3, 319-331.

Luecke, D. (1981). *The relationship manual for couples*. Columbia MD: The Relationship Institute.

Martin, D., & M. Martin (1992). *Stepfamilies in therapy: Understanding systems, assessment, and intervention*. San Francisco, CA: Jossey-Bass.

Meichenbaum, D. (1985). *Stress inoculation training*. NY: Pergamon Press.

National Center for Health Statistics. (1991). Advanced report of final marriage statistics, 1988. *Monthly vital statistics report* (Vol. 40, No. 4, suppl.). Hyattsville, MD: Public Health Service.

Ricci, I. (1980). *Mom's house, dad's house*, NY: Macmillan.

Roskies, E. (1987). *Stress management for the healthy type a*. NY: Guilford.

Sager, C. et al. (1983). *Treating the remarried family*. NY: Brunner/Mazel.

Satir, V. (1972). *People Making*. Palo Alto, CA: Science and Behavior Books.

Stanton, G. W. (1986). Preventive intervention with stepfamilies, *Social Work*, May-June: 201-206.

Visher, E., & Visher, R. (1978). Common problems of stepparents and their spouses. *American Journal of Orthopsychiatry*, 48, 252-262.

Visher, E., & R. Visher (1982). *How to win as a stepfamily*. NY: Brunner/Mazel.

Wald, E. (1981). The remarried family: Challenges and promises. NY: *Family Service Association of America*.

Walmyr assessment scales scoring manual. (1992). Tempe, AZ: Walmyr Publishing Co.

Wertkin, R. A. (1985). Stress-inoculation training: Principles and application. *Social Casework*, 66, 10, 611-616.

Willson, B. F., & Clarke, S. C. (1992). Remarriages: A demographic profile, *Journal of Family Issues*, Vol. 13, No. 2, 123-141.

Pilgrimage:
An Extension of the Social Work Agen.
One Response in Social Artistry
by Families to Modernity

Kris Jeter

SUMMARY. The objective of this paper is to illuminate the functions of pilgrimage in the lives of individuals, families, and communities across cultures and millennia. To date, pilgrimage has been unheralded and neglected by social scientists and human service providers. Yet, it is a powerful process for maintaining the psyche and physical well-being of people. Family building and nurturing is another consequence of pilgrimage.

I consider pilgrimages to be innovative social programs in which the social artist can succeed. In this analytic essay, I describe how pilgrimage actually extends the two major aims of social work professionals: one-to-one intervention and social reform. I describe pilgrimages by Sephardic, Oriental, and religious Jews in Israel; focus is on the Moroccan Jews in particular.

INTRODUCTION

Almost two thousand years ago in the Galilee of Israel, there lived a kindly and intelligent rabbi; he worked hard translating

Kris Jeter is Principal, Beacon Associates, LTD., Inc., a Social Research and Consultation Firm.

[Haworth co-indexing entry note]: "Pilgrimage: An Extension of the Social Work Agenda; One Response in Social Artistry by Families to Modernity." Jeter, Kris. Co-published simultaneously in *Marriage & Family Review* (The Haworth Press, Inc.) Vol. 21, No. 1/2, 1995, pp. 157-179; and: *Exemplary Social Intervention Programs for Members and Their Families* (ed: David Guttmann, and Marvin B. Sussman) The Haworth Press, Inc., 1995, pp. 157-179. Multiple copies of this article/chapter may be purchased from The Haworth Document Delivery Center [1-800-3-HAWORTH; 9:00 a.m. - 5:00 p.m. (EST)].

157

have children, thus increasing the segment of the population who have a higher education and status.

Return to ancient pilgrimages indigenous to the varied ethnic groups of Singapore may be preferable to imitating the Western technology of matchmaking. Pilgrimage, the ritual conducted in family and community for expressing thankfulness and intentions may well be a superior way to meet not only one's mate, but to acknowledge stages of the life cycle and stress of societal events. Pilgrimage may well be an innovative, albeit age-old social program that extends the mission of contemporary social service agencies.

CHALLENGE

Social work as a profession began with the introduction of the English Poor Law of 1601 (Dolgoff and Feldstein, 1984). Social workers were charged to ascertain that public funds were not being exploited by recipients. The language of this Elizabethan law did indicate that the community was responsible for its citizens. However, the causes of poverty were ignored.

In the nineteenth century, the Charity Organization Societies in England began to develop a program of social work with two aims (Austin, 1992). The first aim was personal intervention. "Friendly visitors" observed the families in their homes and provided moral lectures along with welfare assistance. The victim was blamed for the impoverished condition. Nevertheless, the friendly visitors were the originators of casework methodology. The second aim of professional social work was to recast the community and restructure the law.

In the twentieth century, with the increasing professionalization of social work, two major theories, based on the aims of social work practice, unfolded (Austin, 1992). The first theory is that welfare recipients are responsible for their own behavior. Social workers are to be therapists trained and skilled in the appropriate use of psychological intervention techniques with their clients. The second theory is that problems in society are caused by modernity. The government is to address, solve, and prevent social problems. Social workers are to conduct research and influence public policy.

The discipline and practice of social work has and continues to develop in response to ever-changing modernity. Medical research increases life spans. Population is a pressing problem for the world. The economy administered by state governments is based on consumption of goods produced by immense corporations using high technology. The disposition of means and capital is far from being fair. The majority of the population live in urban mega-centers; rural extended kinship ties are broken. Knowledge bases multiply and micro-specialize by the minute. The instantaneous dissemination of news, music videos, soap operas, commercials, and game shows homogenizes the world's peoples.

A worst case scenario for bureaucratic social work follows. Social programs planned, administered, and provided by professionals are effective until demand outweighs availability of services and resources. Clients feel that they are considered to be statistics, not humans. Professionals label the clients as deficient malfunctioning beings who need increased formal, more expensive intervention. Mutual contact is lessened. Conviction in one's abilities and satisfaction in one's life decreases. The old service ways are insufficient to meet the rapidity of ideological, political, and social change.

Innovative social programs rely on the concepts of former times. Professional social workers are simply consultants stimulating thought, communication, and action. Persons willing to be "social service extenders" are welcomed and embraced. John E. Horojai, Thomas Walz, and Patrick R. Connolly (1977, p. 176) defined social service extenders as persons who are *not* paid professional or paraprofessional social workers who encounter a problem in the community and engage the community to enact solutions. I use the word, extension, to describe nonprofessional actions which, nevertheless, augment and promote the aims of social work.

Extension of the social work aims may be furthered by a variety of individuals. Marvin B. Sussman (1991) has introduced the term and described the role of "the social artist." The social artist is a person with an integrated emotional, intellectual, physical, and spiritual system deepened in conscious, and committed to provide consultation, guidance, and leadership in changing paradigms, values, legislation, laws, and structures of society.

My interest in social work is deeply rooted in my youth. At age nine, my family moved from a prairie town of entrepreneurs to a mountain village of coal miners whose coal was no longer desired. The young adults moved to the big cities. The folks who remained held their bodies and souls together with the band-aids of welfare dollars. My life has forever been influenced. I have devoted my life to the education and civil rights of people of all cultural, economic, and social status. I anticipate that the majority of professionals who work in social work have a story in their past that has profoundly influenced their choice, and more important, their philosophy and practice of a career.

There have never been and will never be enough band-aids of welfare dollars. We are intensely challenged to identify and extend extant innovative social programs. I believe that pilgrimage may well extend two major aims of social work professionals: one-to-one intervention and social reform.

My interest in pilgrimages as a means to enhance the practice of social work is based on pilgrimage experience while on a number of journeys to the Middle East: Egypt, Israel, Jordan, Syria, and Turkey. After intensive reading, I sought colleagueship. Issachar Ben-Ami of Hebrew University has kindly mentored me in this work. During the springs of 1992 and 1993, I was a participant/observer at eight sites in Israel before, during, and after the pilgrimage. Below, I list each the name of each pilgrimage in Hebrew and English, its date on the Hebrew calendar, and site(s).

Mimouna, death date of Maimonides, 22 Nisan, Elijah's Cave, Haifa

Yom Ha'Atzmaut, Israel Independence Day, 5 Iyar, Tomb of Baba Sali, Neti Vot and Elijah's Cave, Haifa

Pesah Sheni, Second Passover, 15 Iyar, Tomb of Rabbi Meir Baal Haness, Rabbi Meir, the Miracle Worker, Tiberias

Lag B'Omer, Thirty-third Day of Omer Counting after Passover and Scholar's Day, 18 Iyar, Traditional Tombs of Rabbi Shimon Bar Yochai, Simon son of Yochai, Mt. Meron and Shimon haZaddick, Simon the Righteous, Jerusalem

Hillula, Kaf-heh B'Iyar, 25 Iyar, death date of Rabbi Chaim Chouri, Tomb of Rabbi Chaim Chouri, Beersheba

> *Shavuot*, 6 Sivan, Feast of Seven Weeks after Passover, HaKo-
> tel (The Western or Wailing Wall) and King David's
> Tomb, Jerusalem
> *Rosh Chodesh Eve*, day before the new moon and new month,
> Rachel's Tomb, Bethlehem
> *Night before the New Moon and the Full Moon*, Tomb of Dan,
> Eshta'ol.

In addition, I visited over sixty other tombs. Each tomb, each celebration has its own flavor and personality.

MOROCCAN JEWS

> The veneration of saints is a universal phenomenon: it passes
> like a thread through all religions, both monotheistic and non-
> monotheistic. In this phenomenon not only do religious as-
> pects come to expression, but also, historical sociological,
> folklorist, economic, cultural, political.
>
> –Issachar Ben-Ami
> *Folk Veneration of Saints Among the Moroccan Jews*

The history of Morocco has been an interplay between Berbers,
the indigenous people of the mountains; the Arabs of the plains; the
French and Spanish in the imperial cities of Fez, Marrakesh,
Méknes, and Rabat; the Oriental Jews of the country; and the Sephardi Jews of the coastal cities. Over the millennium, the Moroccan population experienced benign or repressive rule, interspersed
with invasions, forced conversions, plagues, and famine.

Raphael Patai (1986) has written the history and mythology of
Moroccan Jews. Cemetery inscriptions indicate Oriental Jews lived
in Morocco from at least the second century C.E. Sephardi Jews
fled Spain in 1391 and 1492, and from Portugal in 1496 and many
immigrated to Morocco. In 1862, the Alliance Israélite Universelle
started schools in Morocco; Jewish girls and boys were taught
Hebrew, Arabic, French, and religion. This education effort increased literacy, idealized European sophistication, and further separated Jews from the less educated gentiles. At the same time, the

mellahs or Jewish quarters of cities were the most densely popu-
lated of all quarters; the average space per person was two square
meters.

Mythology provides us with a very interesting cultural mirror.
Raphael Patai's (1983) analysis of Jewish Moroccan folklore de-
picts Jewish and Muslim characters to be self-assured. Both speak
and act forthrightly. Muslims come to the rabbi and ask for counsel
and blessings.

With the establishment of Israel in 1948, the withdrawal of the
French from Morocco, and the unstable strides toward Moroccan
independence, terrorist acts against Jews increased. Jews immigrated abroad, 200,000 going to Israel. Although a Jewish community did remain, the economics of the country was negatively
affected by the leave-taking of a people who had primarily acted as
intermediaries between the varied cultural groups. In 1976, King
Hassan invited Jews to immigrate back to Morocco, offering full
citizenship. Few, if any, Israelis moved back to Morocco.

In accordance with the pattern for immigrants in general, Jewish
families who chose to move from Morocco realized that the
struggles would be most significant for the adults. In time, they
knew that the benefits would be highest for the children. However,
the Moroccans faced many challenges to family life.

With the mass migration to Israel of the majority of Jews in
Morocco, primary concern was on preservation of Moroccan
Jewery. Extended kin were separated into nuclear families and
moved to varied parts of Israel. State planners divided and dis-
persed families geographically so that war or natural catastrophe
could not eliminate an entire bloodline. In the assimilation process,
old traditions became suspect or were forgotten and ignored.

For as long as 2,500 years, Oriental Jews and, for as long as
1,500 years, Sephardi Jews have lived among Arabs. There have
been similarities to varied degrees, according to clan and geograph-
ic place, in the marital customs of Jews and Muslims. For instance,
a twelve-year old female might be legally married so that she can
actually "grow up" with her husband's family in his home. Muslim
law allows a man to have four wives if he can support them. Thus,
on infrequent occasion, a Muslim or Jewish man living in an Arab
country could be a bigamist.

In Israel, laws were quickly passed to address these rare familial customs, strange, indeed, to Ashkenazi. In 1950, the Knesset passed a law setting the minimum age of marriage for women at 17 years. A year later, polygamy was outlawed (Patai, 1953, 324-6). Other laws and practices influenced Moroccan families. Compulsory schooling and military service integrated youth. More and more marriages were intermarriages. Moreover, the worldwide trend for Westernization has further eroded the kinship network.

At risk, in the last century especially, have been the stable kin groups of Moroccan Jews, assaulted in Morocco and then in Israel by the interplay of politics and modernity. Within the early years of immigration, the need for innovative social programs for Moroccan Jewish families in Israel became evident. Devout religious as well as politically active Israelis from Morocco reinstated an age old tradition, pilgrimage to tombs, which has facilitated, I believe, at least two aims of formal social work: one-to-one intervention and social reform.

PILGRIMAGES TO TOMBS

The saint is subordinated to his Essence;
A devotee, but in the Way of Essence.
His work arrives at its end
When its beginning arrives again at its end.

–Shabistari (Shah)

Within the geography of the Middle East, from Morocco to Iran, domed tombs of Jewish, Christian, and Muslim saints appear on the landscape. There is always a yearning for the archetype of home, a remembrance of a sweetness of childhood, a glorification of known and unknown ancestors, a wish for far-reaching intergeneration connection, a desire to be blessed, if only for a moment, by saints, intermediaries to the most Powerful. Over millennia, the tomb became a sacred space for kin and strangers to gather and request the kind of intervention of a beloved and respected saintly human.

The tradition of tomb building and saint veneration is ancient. The Hebrew Scriptures indicate that Abraham had a vision of the Garden of Eden within a cave. Abraham purchased the cave for 400 silver shekels, the equivalent of two years of labor (Levy,), to be the burial site for his family. Today, the Cave of Machpelah, covered by a tremendous Herodian building, is the traditional burial site of Adam and Eve, Abraham and Sarah, Isaac and Rebecca, along with Jacob and Leah. The Cave of Machpelah is also called *Haram el-Khalil,* in Arabic, the Shrine of the Beloved God (Murphy-O'Connor, 1986).

Early Christians provide travel accounts of their pilgrimages to Israel. The Roman mother and daughter, Paula and Eustochium in 386 CE, as well as Arculfus, a bishop of Gaul in 670 CE attest to the presence of tombs and the veneration of the matriarchs and patriarchs by Jews and Christians.

Mohammed said, "The most beautiful tomb is one that vanishes from the face of the earth" (Burckhardt, 1976). However, the old tradition was maintained and between the twelfth and fourteenth centuries enhanced by Seljuk rulers building mausoleums for themselves and disciples constructing tombs for Sufi saints. The *wali-Allah,* "friend of God," is considered to be a live mediator for the human with God. Muslims seek the saint's *barakah* or blessing.

Issachar Ben-Ami (1981) and Raphael Patai (1986) have written on the cross-veneration of saints by Jews, Christians, and Muslims. Throughout the year, pilgrims visit tombs of saints when they want to express a personal, familial, or social need and pilgrims participate in annual celebrations.

Each year, (Reeves, 1993) Muslims celebrate the *mulidilia* at the tomb on the birthday of the *wali.* (*Mulid* means the happy anniversary of birth and *mulidores* is the past tense for devotion.) The celebration is joyous and akin to the Jewish *hillula.*

In the Oriental and Sephardic tradition, the matriarchs and righteous women are called *zaddikot* and *zaddikim.*

Jews participate in the *hillula.* The word, *hillula* (plural *hilluloth*), is derived from the Aramaic and means "wedding celebration" (Weingrod, 1990, p. 11). The death date is celebrated because it is believed that *zaddikot* and *zaddikum* experience *mitat neshikah,* death by a divine kiss. The soul, kissed by God, rejoins its wellspring (Deuteronomy 34:5; Jacobs, 1990, 111). According to mystical writings, this is an auspicious time to study the Torah, contemplate one's life, to pray, to celebrate the life of the *zaddik.* Perhaps, on this anniversary of the righteous person's death by a divine kiss, the pilgrim can court, and maybe marry her or his own soul.

The pilgrimage to the tombs, the celebration of the *hillula* have, I contend, actually become innovative social programs for Moroccan Jews in Israel. As discussed below, the tradition of pilgrimage draws kin together into an atmosphere where one-to-one intervention and social action can take place.

ONE-TO-ONE INTERVENTION

> . . . I believe that we shall no longer spill so much blood and waste so much time on problems of methodology (i.e., Rankian versus Freudian psychology; counseling versus case work) which really are meaningless, and falsely assume that there is but one road to salvation . . . We are going to recapture more and more of the warmth [and personal approach] which we had a generation ago in family work, some of which we have lost in this search for more and more scientific and objective treatment processes.

> –Maurice B. Hexter

Contemporary social workers have ever expanding case loads and paper work. Time to listen with empathy, to talk and work with each client is, indeed, an unheard of luxury. Professionals burn out, attempting to express human concern in an often less-than-human bureaucracy full of governmental red tape. Pilgrimages are times set aside on the calendar in which the person elects to commune with her or his self, family, other pilgrims, and nature. The saints are considered to be proficient in facilitating miracles. Each person is met with an open heart; each step taken is known to be a step on sacred land. Anything is possible in this holy atmosphere.

There is preliminary preparation for a pilgrimage. Religious persons may go to the mikvah, the ritual bath. Candles, arak, soft drinks, cookies, candies, and crackers are purchased. Egg dishes and couscous may be cooked ahead and pastries baked. Fresh fruit and herbs may be picked from the garden. Silver platters are brought for serving.

The trip, itself, may well lead to personal exchange and one-to-one intervention. A number of pilgrimages occur on or near religious holidays when there is no public transportation. Moreover, the tombs tend to be "off the beaten track." Thus, pilgrims arrange rides with friends and kin or hitchhike. I was blessed to have the use of a rental car and was asked to or offered to give rides to pilgrims. Our conversations were most reflective and intimate. Pilgrims told me of their intentions and the charge to action they felt they were receiving from their participation in the ritual.

Annually, many kin groups rent buses. In the company of large extended families, pilgrims make pilgrimage from tomb to tomb. The family reunion occurs in sacred space and time.

The tombs are generally in awe-inspiring settings, such as the desert, hills, mountains, and springs. For instance, the tomb of Rabbi Meir Baal Haness is south of Tiberias on a hill overlooking Lake Kinnerit, the Sea of Galilee. The tomb is inside a magnificent new building. The architecture is well designed; the tomb, yeshiva (school), synagogue, and spaces for varied pilgrim activities are united by a circular traffic flow pattern. The tomb itself is in a large domed room. Birds fly freely in an out of the open windows. The birds' songs from their nests in the chandeliers and the view of the Kinnerit Lake heighten reverence for all creation. It is a cool place to be in the summer and warm in the winter.

The tomb is an excellent place for respite care. There is a feeling of calm and peacefulness. Fathers and mothers cradle babies in their arms, kiss them softly, sing gentle tunes. After saying prayers, children quietly play, while kin visit. Single parents attending specifically to one child would often ask me or other pilgrims to keep an eye out on the rest of the family. Respite care is available in a serene environment.

The walk to the tomb itself may be a time for communing with nature, as well as physically invigorating and restorative. For instance, the walk to the traditional tomb of Queen Esther and her uncle, Mordechi, near Barum is a hike up hills and down valleys. Growing among the dense growth of a natural forest, wild flowers bloom, such as the red tears of the Maccabees and yellow rotum. For the infirm, the exercise may be unusual and beneficial to wellness.

It is not uncommon for pilgrims to set up camp for the pilgrimage. The most popular pilgrimage is Lag B'Omer; 300,000 attended in 1992, the 159th consecutive year of celebration. The Abu family led the annual several-mile parade down and up hills from Zfat to Mt. Meron. The Torah from Beit Abu is carried. A number of participants arrive two months ahead of time, so that they have camping sites nearest to the tomb. Generators and other conveniences are set up. Three large video screens permit a view of the bonfire, welcome speech by the Minister of Religious Affairs, and entertainers. There are large parking lots for buses and cars. Fleets of buses transport families from the lots to the camping and tomb areas. A high level of security is present. Two clinics operate with 60 volunteers, four physicians, and two paramedics ("Mt. Meron," 1992).

The site itself is considered to hold the power of generations expressing the spectrum of human hopes and dreams. Three sites, in particular, are associated with particular needs: the tomb of Rabbi Jonathan Ben Uzziel in Amuka for meeting one's mate; Rachel's Tomb in Bethlehem for fertility and protection of children; and Elijah's Cave in Haifa for mental health.

The empathy of matriarch Rachel for human concerns crosses almost 4000 years of time and three religions. Rachel, the beloved wife, experienced the deep yearning for a child. Rachel, the mother who died in childbirth, weeps even today for us, her children. Roman Catholics enter and leave the building, making the sign of the cross and bowing three times. Muslims visit the tomb and pray. Jews tie red cotton cord around the tomb seven times, say prayers, and rewind the cord into a coil. Some people give the cords to friends during times of great adversity. Elders may take the coils to sacred sites, tie cord on the right hand of pilgrims and say a prayer. Believers, especially mothers and children, wear the cord to ward off the evil eye. This belief is based on Jeremiah 31:14-16; here we meet "Rachel weeping for her children."

Elijah's Cave (Vilnay, 1978) has a long reputation for being a site where mental illness is cured. Traditionally, the patient sleeps in the cave for three nights. In the mid-nineteenth century, a newspaper article detailed the cure of an adolescent woman with Torrette Syndrome. One night, while she slept in the grotto, she was blessed with a dream. Elijah and Elisha instructed her to bath in Lake Kinnerit. With this immersion, she regained her health and composure.

Elijah and his cave are considered holy to Jews, Christians, Muslims, and Druze. Jews call the cave the School for the Prophets. Each year, on the fourteenth of June, the Carmelite Order says mass in the cave to honor Elisha, the student of Elijah. Many Christians believe that the Holy Family rested in the cave when they returned from Egypt to Nazareth. Muslims and Druze call Elijah Al Hadar, the green one who is always alive and available to assist humankind. Muslims pray, make vows, and ask for a clipping of hair from an unrelated pilgrim. For centuries, this cave has been ascribed to be the site for miraculous healing and good fortune.

The ritual pilgrimage often contains the following elements. At the entrance to the complex, a vendor may sell ethnic and religious items. It is considered auspicious to purchase an object; the pilgrimage can be remembered and the vendor can in some small part be remunerated for service to the site. Bags of incense are popular purchases; the incense includes cinnamon, cloves, sulfur, white clay and sixteen other ingredients. The directions indicate that it is to be burned on Monday, Thursday, and Friday in order to secure good communication, health, income, and luck. While the incense burns on a plate, the believer steps over it seven times, passes it over the head seven times, and inhales three times.

Outside the cave, elder women or men may tie red cord blessed at Rachel's Tomb around the right hands of pilgrims, especially women and children. Before entering the cave, everyone covers their heads and Jews touch the mezuzah. Jews from India leave their shoes outside the door. A minyan may be formed and prayers recited in unison. Occasionally, the sounds of "amen" as well as women's twills crescendo.

Individuals may go behind large royal blue or majestic red velvet curtains. Here, the head may be rested upon the right arm which is touching the cave wall. Some persons talk in a conversation with their bosom buddy, Elijah. Others sob, cry, wail, and weep; afterwards, they may lay a cloth down on the cave's floor, nap, and even dream. Catharsis occurs; pilgrims leave refreshed, their stature restored, faces softened.

Blessings may be requested from rabbis and money placed in the palm. Coins are dropped in every collection box. Arak, soft drinks, saltines, sweets, fruits, egg dishes, and couscous are passed around by families to fellow journeyers. Freshly picked hadas, mint, and myrtle may be left at the case for prayer books or given personally to pilgrims. Upon leaving the cave, the mezuzah is touched again. Outside, candles are lit and prayers recited in a special area. The candle (Shalem, 1993) symbolizes the human body; the spirit goes up and the body goes down. Moreover, the soul is attracted to light.

Families may picnic. Some sites have special areas for ritual butchering of sheep and cattle. There may be traditional music and dancing, exchange of jokes, and telling of folktales. The pilgrimage is a ritual of genuine bliss, delight, and enjoyment.

Pilgrimage provides an opportunity for one-to-one intervention. Before the pilgrimage, the individual faces what is most feared, is challenged to assess the present life and consider the future. During the pilgrimage, in community, there is mutual giving. The extended family and fellow pilgrims with a shared history act as a coherent support group. The entire day is set aside for listening to and telling life stories, making social connections and interventions. Resources are recommended. Ritual smooths out all differences. Life can be met bravely, in community, and lived richly. Human relationships are cherished and the human spirit is elevated. Charged by being with empathetic kin and friends in sacred time and space, the pilgrim views life refreshed, with new insights and ideas.

SOCIAL REFORM

Whatever environmental and organizational forces are at play, organizational change is *executed by people* whose action is governed by the meaning these forces have for them, their preferences for one or another outcome, and the intensity with which these preferences are held.

–George Brager and Stephen Holloway

The social work client needs to be known and recognized, to see and be seen, within the context of the community. In Israel, Moroc-

can Jewish pilgrimages have been most instrumental in reaffirming
ethnic pride and activities facilitating social reform. In community,
personal issues loose their gravity when viewed holistically. The
question, "What is our future?" becomes the focal point. Pilgrims
are transported to see their local concerns in the larger pattern of the
human condition. Problems become challenges to be met as if old
friends.

Issachar Ben-Ami (1981) has proposed a three-stage process that
Moroccan Jews have taken in Israel regarding pilgrimage that, I
believe, can also be applied to social reform.

1. After arrival, during the early 1950s pilgrimages were made
   by some new immigrants to conventional sacred sites, such as
   Elijah's Cave and tombs in Mt. Meron, Tiberias, and Zfat. In
   general, most human effort was allocated to survival in a new
   environment with lessened kin support and acculturation, i.e.,
   becoming citizens in an independent Israel.
2. During the late 1950s and early 1960s, groups would meet in
   homes and synagogues on the eve of the death date of a *zaddikot* and *zaddik*, the righteous female or male. Traditions were
   reenacted within a small community. Immigrants settled in Israel and proud of their heritage formed the nucleus for ethnic
   pride and social reform.
3. From the mid 1960s large scale *hilluloth* have developed.
   Many righteous persons were buried in North Africa and with
   the Mass migration, their tombs have been neglected. Issachar
   Ben-Ami (1981) has addressed this issue, writing in particular
   about the remembrance of Rabbi David u-Moshe. Although
   Rabbi David u-Moshe is buried abroad, he is presently vener-
   ated in a house in Zfat in northern Israel and in a synagogue in
   Ashkelon in southern Israel.

Avraham Ben Hayim has devoted his house to the memory of the
zaddik. After listening to Mr. Ben Hayim speak, I told him I felt the
authenticity of his act. He responded, "I tell people that I had a
dream. This they can accept. However, this is not entirely true. I *had*
to build this shrine. There was no question in my mind. I *had* to
build this shrine. I was called to do this." In time, the immigrant
fully feels and expresses cultural knowledge and personal power.

In my observations of religious pilgrimages in America and Europe, participants are overwhelming women. This does not appear to be the case with North African Jewish pilgrimages in Israel. Families–men and women–participate. Adolescents may choose not to participate. However, teenagers attend pilgrimages when they join the military and when they marry and have families.

The reinstatement of the *Mimouna* pilgrimage has been most provocative. The *Mimouna* was celebrated in Morocco and Libya and is most popular today. During Passover week, all leavened products are removed from the house. Muslim neighbors celebrate the end of Passover, bringing leavened breads and pastries to their Jewish friends (Ilsen, 1992). The *Mimouna* is a *hillula* celebration in homage of the anniversary of the death of Rabbi Moses ben Maimon (Patai, 1986, 178), the renowned Spanish physician and philosopher, who is often called Maimonides and Rambam. Written evidence first refers to the *Mimouna* in the eighteenth century (Ben-Ami, 1981). The name itself may be related to the Hebrew word, *emunah*, which means "belief," "faith." The *Mimouna* starts at the first sundown ending Passover week. In North Africa, Jewish youth would join the nightly promenade, prominent in the Mediterranean Sea, only on this night dressed in Arab garb (Goldberg, 1978, 76). Kin and friends would make social calls, sharing holiday food and mahia, and arak. Prayers of thanksgiving and benedictions are recited. The next day, kin would spend the day in nature. Prospective spouses might take the opportunity to look at each other. Marriages were often negotiated and announced during the *Mimouna.*

A small group of politically astute, socially active Moroccan immigrants planned and announced a nation wide *Mimouna.* Local celebrations were to be held at Elijah's Cave, the tomb of Rabbi Choni Hameagel, and other sacred sites. The major celebration would be at the Sachar Park, near the Knesset in Jerusalem. Politicians and the Chief Rabbis speak; celebrities perform. There are exhibits to visit. Families congregate and picnic. The *Mimouna* is a holiday in which everyone wants to be a Moroccan. Harvey Goldberg (1978) has noted that in Morocco, young people during the *Mimouna* would dress as if they were Arab, assume a majority status. Today in Israel, the celebration of the *Mimouna* places Moroccans in the majority status–at least for a day. It is such a success, other ethnic groups have started celebrations: the Kurdish *Seherra-na*, Persian *Ruz-e-begh*, and the Ethiopian *Sigd* (Weingrod, 1990).

There is a full circle between social reform and political action. At two of the five pilgrimages at which I was a participant observer before a national election, laminated prayer cards and audio tapes of political speeches were presented to pilgrims by political parties.

One-to-one intervention and social reform can, in this the context of ethnic traditions can humanize the experience of social welfare and nourish the client emotionally. Pilgrimage may well be the extension of social work in which the aims of the social artist are accomplished.

CONCLUSION

Social action for change in advance is inescapable, unless we are willing to drift along eternally patching up the consequences of social neglect and industrial breakdown.

–Helen Hall,
a pioneer of the settlement house movement 1936

Before the 1980s the primary method utilized to recommend social policy was to deduce the causes of problems by statistical analysis and even manipulation of collected census and survey data. Experimental research conducted to study possible public policy began in the late 1960s with the negative income tax study. Passell (1992) forecasts that United States President Bill Clinton will recommend increased utilization of experiment-based research and evaluation of social programs as the basis for formulating social policy. Perhaps research on rituals and pilgrimages could prove valuable.

In complex societies today, the television talk show has become an extension of social work. It is a secular pilgrimage for the West, albeit physical movement might be limited to pushing the remote control switch from a seat on the sofa. Over the past twenty-five years, talk shows have proliferated from interviews with public personalities to open confessionals for persons describing their life experiences. Hosts may have free or pay-per-minute telephone numbers for listeners to call. Callers' concerns are noted and discussed over the air. The host may act as a therapist. The studio and television audience listens with varied degrees of empathy and engage in a form of network therapy. Publications, self-help groups, press agents, and social action may result. Yet, where is the human contact, the sacred space, the ancient ritual, the sensual delight, the healing nature?

Pilgrimage is an ancient tradition in which each person has the potential to become a social artist. The phenomenon is not limited to one religion or culture. It is cross-cultural. China Galland in *Longing for Darkness* (1990) describes her personal growth during her pilgrimage to sites sacred to the Buddhist goddess, Tara and the Christian Black Madonna. Her description of the two-week walk with thousands of other pilgrims to Our Lady of Czestochowa give us insights into the strong connection between this annual pilgrimage, the Solidarity movement, and Poland's ultimate independence. Edward B. Reeves in *The Hidden Government* (1990) provides us with an anthropological view of the annual pilgrimage to the Tanta Wali complex in the Egyptian delta. The relationship that humans have with the saint are the model for the relationships humans have with each other. As the Egyptian bureaucracy enlarges, clientelism and pilgrimage decrease.

Pilgrimage is an institution with influence often outweighing government edicts. For instance, recently I (Jeter, 1993) discussed pilgrimages by Muslims to ancient Hindu temples, Candi Sukuh and Candi Ceto high in the mountains of central Java. The government, which has made great strides in population control, is concerned about the popularity and power of an ancient fertility ritual. It has erected at the entrance to this fertility temple a ten-foot statue of two fingers, reminding Indonesian pilgrims that families with two children only are best!

During pilgrimage, the entire world opens up; healing is possible, even when a cure is not. The opportunity is presented to start life anew. Everyone has wounds and pains which cannot be hidden. In the context of a pilgrimage, illnesses may or may not be cured; however, healing, the feeling of wholeness, is most possible. Cognitive, emotional, and physical attention is presented to one's self, family, and community. Friends and kin entrust themselves to each other. Shifts in approaches to solving life problems occur because of the intense expression of care, concern, and love. Isolation weakens people; tender communication reassures people, evoking the will to live consciously, mindfully. Healing is recognized as the personal attributes a person brings to the process itself, the inner resources gathered together and utilized.

Pilgrimage may be a process in the amortarium of the social worker. Affective, instructive, material, and networking support is shared in community by family and kin. Pilgrimage promotes psychological and physical health, fosters kinship and friendship ties, encourages equitable sharing of resources, and provides an environment for respite care. While celebrating the miracles of life, pilgrims, in family and community ponder, connect, plan, and work toward solving problems at home. Pilgrims, united and empowered by a common spiritual intention, inspired with courage and fortitude, have succeeded in transforming society to be more equitable.

REFERENCES

Abihssira, Baroukh. (1982). *Le Saint Venere Israel Abihssira Sidna Baba Salé: Bibliographie Détaillée et Documentée.* Netivoth, Israel:_ . (French; translated by author.)

Aradi, Zsolt. (1954). *Shrines to Our Lady around the World.* New York, NY: Farrar, Straus and Young, 63, 64.

Ausubel, Nathan, editor. (1948). *A Treasure of Jewish Folklore.* New York, NY: Crown Publishers.

Austin, Carol D. (1992). "Social Work." Encyclopedia of Sociology. Volume 4. Edited by Edgar F. Borgatta and Marie L. Borgatta. New York, NY: Macmillan Publishing Company, pp. 1979-1984.

Begg, Ean. (1985). *The Cult of the Black Virgin.* Updated Edition. New York, NY: Arkana.

Ben-Ami, Issachar. (1986). "Folklore." *Enclyclorama of Israel.* Jerusalem, Israel: Edition et Diffusion Mondiale. 229-347

Ben-Ami, Issachar. (1981). "Folk veneration of saints among the Moroccan Jews." *Studies in Judaism and Islam* edited by Shelomo Morag, Issachar Ben-Ami, and Norman A. Stillman. Jerusalem: The Magnes Press, the Hebrew University.

Ben-Ami, Issachar. (19 May 1992). Personal Communication. Amuka, Israel.

Brager, George and Stephen Holloway (1978). *Changing Human Service Organizations: Politics and Practice.* New York, NY: The Free Press. 80.

Braslavsky, Joseph. (1954). *Studies in Our Country: Its Past and Remains.* Tel Aviv, Israel: Hakibbutz Hameuhad Publishers.

Burckhardt, Titus. (1976). "Tombs." *Art of Islam: Language and Meaning.* England: World of Islam Festival Publishing Company, Ltd., pp. 93-97.

Campbell, Ena. (1982). "The Virgin of Guadalupe and the Female Self-Image: A Mexican Case History." *Mother Worship: Theme and Variations.* James J. Preston, Editor. Chapel Hill, NC: The University of North Carolina Press, 5-24.

Canaan, Taufik. (1927). *Mohamadean Saints and Sanctuaries in Palestine.* London: Luzac.

Cohen, Erik. (Summer 1983). "Ethnicity and Legitimation in Contemporary Israel." *The Jerusalem Quarterly,* 28, 111-124.

Crapanzano, Vincent. (1975). "Saints, Jnun, and Dreams: An Essay in Moroccan Ethnopsychology." *Psychiatry,* 38, 145-159.

Deshen, Shlomo and Moshe Shokeid. (1974). *The Predicament of Homecoming: Cultural and Social Life of North African Immigrants in Israel.* Ithaca NY: Cornell University Press.

Dictionary of Mary. (1985). New York, NY: Catholic Book Publishing Company.

Dolgoff, Ralph; and Donald Feldstein. (1984). *Understanding Social Welfare,* Second Edition. New York, NY: Longman.

Eastern Regional Conference on Apparitions of the Mother and Her Divine Son. Our Lady of Peace Ministries, Sponsors. (13-14 July 1991). Pittsburgh, PA: A.J. Palumbo Center, Duquesne University.

Eliade, Mircea. (1959). *The Sacred and the Profane.* Translated from the French by Willard R. Trask. New York, NY: Harcourt, Brace and World, Inc.

Fischer Joel. (1973). "Is casework effective: A review." *Social Work,* 18, 5-20.

Galland, China. (1990). *Longing for Darkness: Tara and the Black Madonna; A Ten-Year Journey.* New York, NY: Penguin Books.

Gebara, Ivone and Maria Bingemer. (1989). *Mary: Mother of God, Mother of the Poor.* Translated by P. Berryman. Maryknoll, NY: Orbis Books.

Gibbons, Ann. (26 February 1993). "Empathy and Brain Evolution." *Science,* Volume 259: Number 5099, page 1250-1251.

Goldberg, Harvey. (1978). "The Mimouna and the Minority Status of Moroccan Jews." *Ethnology,* 17, 75-85.

Goldberg, Harvey. (1983). "The Mellahs of Southern Morocco." *The Maghreb Review,* 9, 61-69.

Graves, Robert and Raphael Patai. (1983). *Hebrew Myths: The Book of Genesis.* New York, NY: Greenwich House.

Greenwood, Ernest. (1957). "Attributes of a profession." *Social Work,* 2, 45-55.

Grinnell, Richard. (1981). *Social Work Research and Evaluation.* Itasca, IL: Peacock.

Hall, Helen. (1936). "The consequences of social action for group work agency." *Proceedings of the National Conference on Social Work.* Columbus, OH: National Conference on Social Welfare, 235, 237.

Hexter, Maurice B. (1966). "The Next Twenty-Five Years in Jewish Communal Service." *Trends and Issues in Jewish Social Welfare in the United States,*

1899-1958. Edited by Robert Morris and Michael Freund. Philadelphia, PA: The Jewish Publication Society of America, 606.

Holy Bible. ( ). King James Version. Cleveland, OH: The World Publishing Company.

Horojai, John E., Thomas Walz, and Patrick R. Connolly. (1977). *Working in Welfare: Survival through Positive Action.* Iowa City, IA: University of Iowa School of Social Work.

Ilsen, Eve. (15 March 1992). Persona Communication. Philadelphia, PA.

Jacobs, Louis. (1990). *Holy Living: Saints and Saintliness in Judaism.* Northvale, NJ: Jason Aronson, Inc., p. 111.

Jayakar, Pupul. (1990). *The Earth Mother.* San Francisco, CA: Harper and Row.

Jeter, Kris. (1991). "Hospitality: An Ancient Proponent for the Wider Family." *Marriage & Family Review: Wider Families: New Traditional Family Forms,* 17, 1&2, 135-158.

Jeter, Kris (1990). "Poverty: A Vision for Heterotopic Eyes, A Question of Values." *The Psychotherapy Patient: The Poverty Patient,* 7, 1/2, 141-147.

Jeter, Kris (1993). "Wedding Rings and Take Out Food: Early Human Mobility Ritualized in Later Human Pilgrimage." *Marriage & Family Review: Families on the Move: Migration, Immigration, Emigration, and Mobility, 19, 1/2, 3/4.*

Josephus. (1988). *The Jewish War.* Translated by G.A. Williamson. Revised Edition. New York, NY: Penguin Books.

The Koran Interpreted. (1955). A. J. Arberry, Translator. New York, NY: Macmillan.

Lanboy, Bezelel. (1972). *The Trip to Meron with Pictures of Holy Places.* Originally published in Jerusalem in 1889 under anonymous author. Jerusalem, Israel: P.A.I.H.K. (Hebrew. Rina Ben-Ari, Translator.)

The Letter of Paula and Eustochium to Marcella, About the Holy Places (386 CE). (1889). Aubrey Stewart,Translator. London, Palestine Pilgrims' Text Society.

Levy, Danny. ( ). *Judaism's Oldest City Comes to Life: The Jewish Community of Hebron.* Jerusalem, Israel: David Derovan.

Mauss, Marcel. (1967). *The Gift: Forms and Functions of Exchange in Archaic Societies.* Translated by Ian Cunnison. New York, NY: W. W. Norton and Company.

Meyer, Henry, and Edgar Bogatta. (1959). *An Experiment in Mental Patient Rehabilitation: Evaluating a Social Agency Program.* New York, NY: Russell Sage Foundation.

Meyer, Henry, Edgar Bogatta, and Wyatt Jones. (1965). *An Experiment in Mental Patient Rehabilitation: An Experiment in Social Work Intervention.* New York, NY: Russell Sage Foundation.

McPherson, J.W. (1941). *The Moulids of Egypt (Egyptian Saints-Days).* Cairo: Nile Mission Press.

Moss, Leonard W. and Cappannair, S. (1982). In Quest of the Black Virgin: She is Black because She is Black. *Mother Worship.* Edited by James J. Preston. Chapel Hill, NC: The University of North Carolina Press.

"Mt. Meron." (Thursday 21 May 1992). *The Jerusalem Post.* LX:18058, p. 1.

Murphy-O'Connor, Jerome. (1986). *The Holy Land: An Archaeological Guide from Earliest Times to 1700.* Second Edition. New York, NY: Oxford University Press.

National Association of Social Workers. (1974). *Standards for Social Service Manpower.* Washington, DC: National Association of Social Workers.

Nelsen, Judith C. (1980). *Communication Theory and Social Work Practice.* Chicago, IL: The University of Chicago Press.

Newman, Edward, and Jerry Turem. (1974). "The crisis of accountability." *Social Work,* 19, 5-16.

Nolan, Mary Lee, and Sidney Nolan. (1989). *Christian Pilgrimage in Modern Western Europe.* Chapel Hill, NC: The University of North Carolina Press.

O'Leary, De Lacy Evans. (1937). *The Saints of Egypt.* New York, NY: Macmillan.

Our Ancestors: A Guide for the Sacred Places in the Galilee. (1989). Second edition. Jerusalem, Israel: Committee for the Conservation of the Ancestors' Tombs (Hebrew).

Passell, Peter. (Tuesday, 9 March 1993). "Like a New Drug, Social Programs Are Put to the Test: Use of Controls Helps Put the Science into Social Science." *The New York Times: Science Times,* Vol: CXLII, No. 49, 265, C1, C10.

Patai, Raphael. (1953). *Israel Between East and West: A Study in Human Relations.* Philadelphia, PA: The Jewish Publication Society of America.

Patai, Raphael. (1986). *The Seed of Abraham: Jews and Arabs in Contact and Conflict.* Salt Lake City, UT: University of Utah Press.

Perry, Nicholas and Loreto Echeverria. (1980). *Under the Heel of Mary.* London, England: Routledge.

The Pilgrimage of Arculfus in the Holy Land About the Year A.D. 670. (1889). James Rose Macpherson, Translator. London, England: Palestine Pilgrims' Text Society.

Pincus, Allen, and Anne Minahan. (1970). "Toward a Model for Teaching a Basic First Year Course in Methods of Social Work." *Practice.* New York, NY: Council on Social Work Education.

Preston, James J., Editor. (1982). "New Perspectives on Mother Worship. *Mother Worship: Theme and Variations.* Chapel Hill, NC: The University of North Carolina Press, 333.

Raymond, Frank. (1977). "A changing focus for the profession: Product rather than process." *Journal of Social Welfare,* 4, 9-16.

Reeves, Edward Bradley. (1990). *The Hidden Government: Ritual, Clientelism, and Legitimation in Northern Egypt.* Salt Lake City, UT: University of Utah Press.

Reeves, Edward Bradley. (Thursday, 4 February 1993). Personal Communication. Morehead, KY: Morehead State University.

Reeves, Edward Bradley. (1984). *The Wali Complex at Tanta, Egypt: An Ethnographic Approach to Popular Islam.* Ann Arbor, MI: University Microfilms International.

Richmond, Mary. (1917). *Social Diagnosis.* New York, NY: Russell Sage Foundation.

Rothman, Jack, John L. Erlich, and Joseph G. Teresa. (1976). *Promoting Innovation and Change in Organizations and Communities: A Planning Manual.* New York, NY: John Wiley and Sons, Inc.

Shabistari. (1970). "The Saint and Essence." *The Way of the Sufi.* Idries Shah. New York, NY: E. P. Dutton, 249.

Shalem, Yisrael. (1991). "Amuka, Rabbi Yonatan Ben Uziel." *Safed.* Safed, Israel: Safed Regional College, Bar Ilan University. 46-47.

Shalem, Yisrael. (1993). Personal Communication. Zfat, Israel.

Sussman, Marvin B. (1991). *Advanced School for Social Artistry.* Newark, DE: The Possible Society and Pamona, NY: The Foundation for Mind Research.

Turner, Victor and Edith Turner. (1978). *Image and Pilgrimage in Christian Culture.* New York, NY: Columbia University Press.

Weingrod, Alex. (1990). *The Saint of Beersheba.* Albany, NY: State University of New York Press.

Vilnay, Zev. (1973). *Legends of Jerusalem.* The Sacred Land. Volume I. Philadelphia, PA: The Jewish Publication Center of America.

Zimdars-Swartz, Sandra L. (1991). *Encountering Mary from La Salette to Medjugorje.* Princeton, NJ: Princeton University Press.

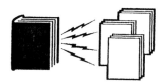

Haworth
DOCUMENT DELIVERY
SERVICE

This new service provides a single-article order form for any article from a Haworth journal.

- *Time Saving:* No running around from library to library to find a specific article.
- *Cost Effective:* All costs are kept down to a minimum.
- *Fast Delivery:* Choose from several options, including same-day FAX.
- *No Copyright Hassles:* You will be supplied by the original publisher.
- *Easy Payment:* Choose from several easy payment methods.

Open Accounts Welcome for . . .
- Library Interlibrary Loan Departments
- Library Network/Consortia Wishing to Provide Single-Article Services
- Indexing/Abstracting Services with Single Article Provision Services
- Document Provision Brokers and Freelance Information Service Providers

---

MAIL or *FAX* THIS ENTIRE ORDER FORM TO:

Attn: **Marianne Arnold**
Haworth Document Delivery Service
The Haworth Press, Inc.
10 Alice Street
Binghamton, NY 13904-1580

or FAX: (607) 722-1424
or CALL: 1-800-3-HAWORTH
(1-800-342-9678; 9am-5pm EST)

PLEASE SEND ME PHOTOCOPIES OF THE FOLLOWING SINGLE ARTICLES:
1) Journal Title: _____

   Vol/Issue/Year:_____Starting & Ending Pages:_____
Article Title:_____
_____

2) Journal Title: _____

   Vol/Issue/Year:_____Starting & Ending Pages:_____
Article Title:_____
_____

3) Journal Title: _____

   Vol/Issue/Year:_____Starting & Ending Pages:_____
Article Title:_____
_____

4) Journal Title: _____

   Vol/Issue/Year:_____Starting & Ending Pages:_____
Article Title:_____
_____

(See other side for Costs and Payment Information)

COSTS: Please figure your cost to order quality copies of an article.

1. Set-up charge per article: $8.00
   ($8.00 × number of separate articles) _____

2. Photocopying charge for each article:

   1-10 pages: $1.00 _____

   11-19 pages: $3.00 _____

   20-29 pages: $5.00 _____

   30+ pages: $2.00/10 pages _____

3. Flexicover (optional): $2.00/article _____

4. Postage & Handling: US: $1.00 for the first article/
   $.50 each additional article _____

   Federal Express: $25.00 _____

   Outside US: $2.00 for first article/
   $.50 each additional article _____

5. Same-day FAX service: $.35 per page _____

   GRAND TOTAL: _____

METHOD OF PAYMENT: (please check one)

❑ Check enclosed   ❑ Please ship and bill. PO # _____
(sorry we can ship and bill to bookstores only! All others must pre-pay)

❑ Charge to my credit card: ❑ Visa;   ❑ MasterCard;   ❑ American Express;

Account Number:_____ Expiration date:_____

Signature: ✗_____ Name: _____

Institution: _____ Address: _____

City: _____ State:_____ Zip:_____

Phone Number: _____ FAX Number: _____

MAIL or *FAX* THIS ENTIRE ORDER FORM TO:

Attn: **Marianne Arnold**
Haworth Document Delivery Service
The Haworth Press, Inc.
10 Alice Street
Binghamton, NY 13904-1580

or **FAX:** (607) 722-1424
or **CALL:** 1-800-3-HAWORTH
(1-800-342-9678; 9am-5pm EST)